Pass the
MRCPsych
(Parts I and II)

Pass the MRCPsych

(Parts I and II)

All the techniques you need

Christopher Williams
Peter Trigwell
David Yeomans

W.B. Saunders Company Ltd
London   Philadelphia   Toronto   Sydney   Tokyo

W.B. Saunders Company Ltd
24–28 Oval Road
London NW1 7DX

The Curtis Center
Independence Square West
Philadelphia, PA 19106-3399, USA

Harcourt Brace & Company
55 Horner Avenue
Toronto, Ontario M8Z 4X6, Canada

Harcourt Brace & Company, Australia
30–52 Smidmore Street
Marrickville, NSW 2204, Australia

Harcourt Brace & Company, Japan
Ichibancho Central Building, 22-1 Ichibancho
Chiyoda-ku, Tokyo 102, Japan

A catalogue record for this book is available from the British Library

ISBN 0-7020-2066-4

Typeset by Keystroke, Jacaranda Lodge, Wolverhampton
Printed and bound in Great Britain by Hartnolls Limited, Bodmin, Cornwall

Contents

Part II: The written exams

Chapter 3   Multiple choice question technique (MCQs)   19
David Protheroe and Chris Williams

Chapter 4   The short answer question paper (SAQs)   31
Peter Trigwell

Chapter 5   Essay technique   47
David Yeomans

Part III   The Clinical Exam

Contributors

Dr Christopher Williams BSc, MB ChB, MMedSc, MRCPsych
Lecturer/Honorary Senior Registrar in Psychiatry, St James's University Hospital, Beckett Street, Leeds LS9 7TF, UK

Dr Peter Trigwell MB ChB, MMedSc, MRCPsych
Senior Registrar in Psychiatry, High Royds Hospital, Menston, Leeds LS29 6AQ, UK

Dr David Yeomans BSc, MB ChB, MMedSc, MRCPsych
Consultant Psychiatrist, Somerset House, Manor Lane, Shipley BD18 3BP, UK

Dr Kevin Appleton MB ChB, MRCPsych
Registrar/Tutor in Psychiatry, St James's University Hospital, Beckett Street, Leeds LS9 7TF, UK

Dr David Protheroe MB ChB, MMedSc, MRCPsych
Senior Registrar in Psychiatry, St James's University Hospital, Beckett Street, Leeds LS9 7TF, UK

Foreword
Professor A.C.P. Sims

The gist of this highly readable and accessible book is how to make the most of what you already have. There are many manuals across all areas of life that aim to take you as you are and help you to make the best of it; this does just that for the partly trained psychiatrist. It is not intended to teach facts but to help candidates present what they know with precision and lucidity. It has been developed from a highly successful course for MRCPsych candidates – both in numbers clamouring to attend the course and an excellent pass rate.

The MRCPsych examination comes in the middle of the training period for a consultant psychiatrist in the United Kingdom and Ireland. Appropriate attitudes, specialist knowledge and therapeutic skills should have already been acquired by that stage, whilst the ability to manage a service, lead a clinical team, undertake psychiatric research and specialise within psychiatry generally comes later. Any question one might have concerning the ultimate usefulness of a work that solely aims to help the candidate over the hurdle of the examination is quickly dispelled: despite its title, this book clearly does more than that. It encourages clarity of thought, marshalling of the factual information that the trainee psychiatrist already has, and expression of facts and opinions in terms that are comprehensible to candidate and examiner alike. For this reason it does not only contribute to passing the examination but also assists in the transition from a junior doctor studying psychiatry to an able and therapeutically effective trained psychiatrist. I would, therefore, commend *Pass the MRCPsych* not only to candidates for the examination but also to their teachers, clinical tutors and educational supervisors.

Andrew Sims, Professor of Psychiatry, University of Leeds.
Immediate Past President of the Royal College of Psychiatrists.
May 1995

Introduction

Clinical competence and passing the Membership Examinations of the Royal College of Psychiatrists are the most visible criteria by which trainees progress up the career ladder in psychiatry. Taking the exams is costly in both financial and personal terms. To pass requires a very significant amount of work and commitment.

This book is not a "crammer" book of key facts for the exam. You will find that very few factual pieces of information are presented. Instead, it will help you to present the information that you have learned elsewhere (whether from formal revision, everyday psychiatric practice or other sources) in a professional and structured way. Even very good clinicians with a strong factual knowledge fail the exams because of poor technique. This book will help you use your knowledge and experience effectively to enable you to pass. At the same time, we hope to help you develop the skills of a good psychiatrist; someone who can manage their time, think quickly and efficiently, and present themselves professionally in exam and interview situations.

The book is divided into three sections. The first section (Preparing for the exam) is intended to help those who are thinking about applying to take either Part of the exam, and are wanting to find out more about the content of the exam. It will also help you think about your learning and revision strategy. The second and third sections of the book cover the written and the clinical parts of the exams, respectively.

We hope that you will find our book helpful. In producing any book such as this, many other people are always involved. We wish to acknowledge the help and support of Dr John Holmes, Dr Peter Elwood and Dr David Thompson, Dr Tony Zigmond, Dr Keith Rix and Professor Sims in particular for their help and ideas in developing the course content. This is much appreciated.

Finally, but most importantly, we wish to thank Alison, Amanda, and Frances for their support and understanding during the writing of this book. Without this it would not have been possible.

Chris Williams, Peter Trigwell, David Yeomans
September 1995

Part I

Preparing for the exam

Chapter 1

Important practical and preparation issues

David Yeomans and Peter Trigwell

STRUCTURE OF THE MRCPsych PARTS I AND II

Part I

- A paper of 50 multiple choice questions (MCQs). Each question has five stems. The MCQ covers descriptive and explanatory psychopathology, methods of clinical assessment in psychiatry, basic clinical psychopharmacology and basic neurosciences. This paper is marked using **negative marking**, so that a mark is subtracted for every wrong response you make. It is therefore important to judiciously decide whether to respond with True, False or Don't Know responses. It is theoretically possible to know the subject very well and answer 74% of questions correctly, and yet still only score 48% as a result of negative marking. This emphasises the need for effective exam technique on this paper.

- Clinical examination, as outlined in Chapter 3. You will have 1 hour with the patient and then be examined on the case for 30 minutes. The Part I clinical exam includes the assessment of patients, but excludes clinical management.

Each part of the exam is marked separately and given a score between 0 and 10. In the Part I examination, a bare pass (4 out of 10) in the MCQ can be compensated for by a good pass (7 out of 10 or more) in the clinical examination. The clinical must, however, be passed in order to pass the Part I exam overall.

Part II

- A paper of 50 MCQs on clinical psychiatry (negative marking).
- A paper of 50 MCQs on "basic sciences" (negative marking). Both MCQ papers are combined to give an overall mark.
- A paper of 20 short answer questions (SAQs).
- Essay paper. This covers both General Adult Psychiatry and also the subspecialities (Child and Adolescent Psychiatry, Forensic Psychiatry, Mental Handicap, Psychiatry of the Elderly, and Psychotherapy).
- Clinical examination. This is made up of two sections, the "long case" **patient assessment** (1 hour with the patient, and 30 minutes with the examiners) and the **patient management problems** (PMPs) (lasting 30 minutes).

The Part II exam is marked so that scores are given between 0 and 20 for each part of the exam. The clinical examination **must be passed** to be successful in the exam. Candidates who obtain a bare fail in the "long case" section of the clinical examination (8 out of 20) can, however, make this up by obtaining a good mark (14 out of 20 or above) in the PMPs, and vice versa.

In the clinical examinations and in the essay, 10 out of 20 is a pass. In the SAQ paper, the pass mark is determined by the difficulty of the paper, and therefore by comparison with the scores of your peers.

All parts of the MRCPsych exams are outlined in the relevant chapters of this book. For more detail, see *Content of the MRCPsych Examinations* which will be sent to you when you apply to sit the exams. It is also very important to obtain the up-to-date College Syllabus in order to find out what areas of knowledge you will be expected to have. It is surprisingly rare for people to send off for this syllabus. In a recent survey of 35 candidates approaching the Part I and Part II exams, less than 10 had obtained the syllabus 6 weeks before the exam. Not one of these candidates would ever dream of attempting the driving test without reading the Highway Code in order to find out what knowledge was necessary!

APPLYING TO SIT THE EXAMS

Timing is important. When is a good time to take the exam?

* For the **Part I MRCPsych**, you must have the equivalent of 1 year's full-time psychiatric training in Adult General Psychiatry before you are eligible. Six months of this experience may be in Psychiatry of the Elderly. You may have between two and four attempts at the exam, over the equivalent of 3 years full-time approved psychiatric training (see *Handbook*

for Inceptors and Trainees in Psychiatry,
available from The Royal College of
Psychiatrists, for full details).

- In order to enter the **Part II MRCPsych** you must
  have the equivalent of 3 year's full-time training
  in psychiatry or 2 year's training plus 1 year of
  approved General Medicine (including
  subspecialities), or 1 year of General Practice,
  or 1 year of full-time research. All training posts
  must be approved by the Royal College and
  details are given in the *Handbook for Inceptors
  and Trainees in Psychiatry.* You are allowed five
  attempts at the Part II exam.

Before taking the exams you will need to save money, plan your
revision, and find two "sponsors". One must be your clinical tutor
and the other a consultant with whom you have worked for at least
4 months during the year prior to the date of application. You must
request application forms from the College, submit these **on time**
with the appropriate fee, and revise. You will have to juggle the
demands this places on you with the time you devote to your
family, friends, and leisure activities. One of the authors put off his
Part I application in order to finish decorating his house. Do what
is right for you.

The deadline for getting your application in is surprisingly early;
you need to request the forms from the College several months in
advance. It is not uncommon for candidates to "miss the boat"
– book early to avoid disappointment and increased stress.

PREPARATION

Once you have decided when to take the exam, immediately work
out a **timetable** for revision. This can inspire increased motivation
to work as you can see just what work needs to be done, and what

areas need to be covered. It will also help to keep you on target for the exam if you stick to your timetable. Most people assign a period of 2–3 months for revision for Part I, and 3–6 months for Part II. It is helpful to work consistently, e.g. 2 hours a night, but be flexible to allow for relaxation, on-call commitments, and other occasions. Many candidates find it helpful to decide upon a day each week when they will definitely **not** revise. Having regular breaks helps to maintain commitment the rest of the time. Remember to continue to have at least some social and "fun" activities. These will be a useful antidote to work.

It may help to structure your revision timetable by following one of the major textbooks. You probably need a check-list of the subject areas in the syllabus to ensure that you cover everything required. It is useful to steadily build up a selection of stock answers for the clinical and oral exams and prepare essays and short answers for MRCPsych Part II.

PRACTICE

An **analysis of your learning style**, as described in the next chapter, will shape the way you prepare for the exams. For every candidate without exception, however, **practice** is essential. It is important to test yourself regularly throughout the revision period in order to get feedback on your performance. For Part I you will need to practise MCQs and clinical examination and presentation. For Part II you will also need to practise writing structured essays, concise short answers to SAQs and reasoned solutions to patient management problems. All these features should be built into your revision timetable.

Familiarity with the actual exam can only be gained through practice. If you doubt this, consider the performance of a slalom skier who has only ever read books on the subject! Be merciless in your pursuit of exam practice. Ask senior colleagues to listen to your presentations and give feedback. Be critical about their comments and do not take it all to heart. Each person you ask will have a slightly different opinion on what is good and bad about your efforts. With adequate practice you will have built up your confidence in your abilities before you enter the examination room.

MENTAL HEALTH

Examinations cause stress over an extended period. It is worthwhile considering how the process is affecting you. Do you need a break? What about a holiday? Or a night out? What about relaxation, sport, television, meditation? If you do suffer from exam nerves it pays to practice relaxation beforehand. Do this in your mock exams too. Although some people have been known to find anxiolytics helpful, medication should generally be avoided.

Last minute revision is sometimes more of an anxiolytic than an aid to memory. Do it if you have to but a day of rest before the exams can also be therapeutic.

GETTING READY FOR THE EXAM

Make it easy on yourself. Get study leave arranged well in advance and stick to it. Consider a revision course prior to the exam. It is often helpful to take a week off work just before the exam to do final preparations. Do not be persuaded to cover for an absent colleague at the last moment; you have spent too much time, effort and money to let personnel issues get in your way. Give yourself at least one clear day off work before travelling to the exam centre. Find a **decent** place to stay before the exam. Do not skimp on last minute comforts, especially if you can claim expenses (ring Personnel in advance to find out what you are entitled to – some employers pay for revision courses too). Give yourself plenty of time to travel. It is better to arrive 2 hours early than 2 minutes late. If using public transport, consider a back-up route if the service is disrupted. In general, if you start out early enough you can cope with traffic and rail delays. Consider flying longer distances. Pack in advance, take plenty of pencils, erasers, money, lucky charms, etc., and do not rush. In the exam, your personal presentation will earn marks. Dress appropriately. Be polite and courteous to everyone.

STATE OF MIND ON THE EXAM DAY

In order to do well in the exams it helps not to be distracted. Some find it easy to concentrate, but others may need to actively focus on the exam and exclude thoughts of work, home and low confidence. Practise relaxation techniques if this helped during revision. Before the exam starts reassure yourself that all your preparation means you are at an advantage, and with luck you will have already prepared answers to some of the questions that will arise.

AFTER THE EXAM

You will not know how things have gone, though you may feel elated or depressed at your performance. Certain parts of the exam, such as the Basic Sciences MCQ paper in Part II, leave the vast majority of candidates feeling that they have probably failed (although obviously many have not). These feelings may continue for some time. Try to avoid too many post-mortems! Going over your answers again and again in your mind analysing possible mistakes is rarely helpful. A holiday break away may be a good idea.

You have to wait a while for the results. If you pass, well done! If not, then **try again** like many members of the Royal College have had to do before. Use the feedback from examiners and keep working on exam technique. (See Chapter 11: If at first you don't succeed . . . .)

REFERENCES

It is worthwhile obtaining and reading the following Royal College publications:

General Information and Regulations for the MRCPsych Examinations

Handbook for Inceptors and Trainees in Psychiatry.
Past Papers in Psychiatry

These can be obtained from:

Royal College of Psychiatrists
17 Belgrave Square
London SW1X 8PG

Tel. 0171 235 2351

Chapter 2

Learning styles and revision strategies

Peter Trigwell and David Yeomans

It is often believed that success in medical examinations simply depends upon the faithful regurgitation of facts. This is not the whole truth. It is certainly possible to know the facts of a subject very well and still fail the examination. You can significantly improve your exam performance with good technique. Technique refers to your style of **learning** and **preparing**, and then of **presenting** the learnt information to best effect.

LEARNING

Sit back for a moment and consider what you know about how you learn. Do you think that you have a personal learning style? It is very likely that you do, since you have spent at least 20 years in education developing your own methods of study. For example, you probably found that your own lecture notes at university were very different from those of your friends.

The following is a list of questions about learning style. Work through it point by point; it is designed to get you thinking about how you learn.

- Do you revise in a **suitable environment**? (For example, quiet, warm enough, well lit, minimum of disturbance.) How can you **improve** the environment?

- Do you **set goals**? (For example, learn the components of the cranial nerves today and test myself tomorrow.)

- Do you **achieve these goals**?

- Do you **structure your learning**? (For example, according to the Royal College syllabus – see *Handbook for Inceptors and Trainees* .[1]) There is no point revising material for the exam which will never be examined. More importantly, you must not miss out subjects that you will be expected to know about.

- Do you know what **sources of information** you are most comfortable with?

Most people use **a group of small books for Part I revision**, such as those listed below. These books are suggestions only, but reflect the sort of level of knowledge and understanding which are required for this exam:

- *Examination Notes in Psychiatry*[2] or another "core book".

- *Introduction to Psychotherapy*[3].

- *Examination Notes for the MRCPsych Part I*[4] – for neurosciences, etc.

- *Symptoms in the Mind*[5] – for psychopathology.

- *ICD 10*.[6]

It is also worthwhile reading relevant sections of the *British National Formulary* (BNF). This contains an up-to-date summary of current prescribing practice.

For **Part II** you may need to decide early on whether you prefer to comprehensively learn a large, up-to-date text (e.g. *Companion to Psychiatric Studies*[7]), supplemented by some journal papers, or use a mixture of smaller books and rather more journal papers. Do not forget to concentrate on the main areas; these are often overlooked as people become bogged down in the fine detail of more obscure topics. Learn psychology and sociology **early**. These are key areas, particularly for the Basic Sciences MCQ paper, and they take quite some time to revise. You should try and avoid the (common) situation where candidates try to learn these subjects from scratch with only a month or so to go.

- Can you **prioritise**? (For example, learn the common things before the esoteric.)

- Do you **keep the exam in mind while learning**? (So as to spot questions, rehearse stock answers and memorise information in the style appropriate to the exam, e.g. as a short answer – see Chapter 9.)

- **How much information** can you take in at one go? (There is no point staring at a book when your concentration seems to have gone. Taking a break will help to consolidate what you have learned.)

- **How much repetition** do you need? (Does it help to read several accounts from differing books, perhaps followed by a re-read of your own notes to fix those facts in your memory? Alternatively, are you the type of person who prefers to learn just one or two books really well?)

- Do you **use your daily work to help you learn**? (For example, practising enquiring after first rank symptoms. Spending time reflecting on your differential diagnoses, formulations, and management plans. Writing up case notes in exam format.)

- Are you **adequately motivated**? (Try to make this positive, e.g. career progression or self-satisfaction, rather than negative, e.g. coercion, financial loss, or fear and "failure avoidance".) Passing the exam requires commitment.

- **Do you compare yourself with others too much**? (Many candidates seem to delight in upsetting the "opposition" during revision and exams and it is important to have a personal sense of your own abilities. Expect some degree of hysteria on revision courses!)

- Do you **use others to help you learn**? (You must be ruthless in getting appropriate clinical exam practice and feedback from your senior colleagues. It is almost pointless to go into the clinical and oral exams without prior practice.)

- Do you **review your progress**? (Plan and write out a **clear revision timetable**, and try to stick to it so that you do not run out of time.)

Do you work best by yourself, or as part of a group? Many find that a combination of approaches is effective. Consider meeting once weekly for several hours with other colleagues who are doing the exam. This can help you to practise parts of the exam (like MCQs) and clarify difficult areas. Supportive **study groups** like this also encourage you during difficult times, and can introduce an element of competition and fun to your revision.

There are many more aspects which go to make up your personal learning style. Spend time thinking about them and check out with others how they approach the process of revision. Use this information to improve your technique. There are many different but effective techniques available to help your learning. One such is to use *Mind Maps*® to summarise and structure your learning (Appendix 1).

Whatever your style, **do not underestimate how much work there is to do**.

PREPARING

With good preparation you can feel confident that the exam is not going to bring up too many surprises and that you can comfortably cope with any that do arise. When doing the exam, although you will feel some anxiety, good preparation should prevent you being thrown off balance by a difficult question, or at least enable you to function on "auto-pilot" until you regain your equilibrium. If you follow the advice in this book, you will have pre-prepared answers and answering techniques for difficult questions. You will know how to impress examiners by your presentation technique. You will know the ins and outs of the exam structure and how it is marked. You will know what is expected of you. All this will help reduce your anxiety and improve your exam performance.

PRESENTING INFORMATION

The following chapters (3 to 11 inclusive) will address the best way to present yourself, and the information you will have learnt, in each individual section of the MRCPsych Part I and Part II examinations. For the past few years, the authors of this book have run The Leeds MRCPsych Examination Technique Course on a biannual basis. Feedback from those attending the course has been extremely good. Many candidates have benefited from the techniques which are taught, and which are now documented in this book. They have improved their exam performance and have successfully passed the exams when employing these techniques. We hope that this will also be the case for you. Please read on.

REFERENCES

[1] Royal College of Psychiatrists, *Handbook for Inceptors and Trainees*, Royal College of Psychiatrists, 17 Belgrave Square, London SW1X 8PG (Tel. 0171 235 2351).

[2] J. Bird and G. Harrison, *Examination Notes in Psychiatry*, 2nd edn, Wright, Bristol, 1987.

[3] D. Brown and J. Pedder, *Introduction to Psychotherapy*, Routledge, London, 1989.

[4] B. Puri and J. Sklar, *Examination Notes for the MRCPsych Part I*, Butterworths, London, 1989.

[5] A. C. P. Sims, *Symptoms in the Mind. An Introduction to Descriptive Psychopathology*, 2nd edn, W. B. Saunders, London, 1995.

[6] World Health Organization, *The ICD10 Classification of Mental and Behavioural Disorders*, WHO, Geneva, 1992.

[7] R. E. Kendell and A. K. Zealley, *Companion to Psychiatric Studies*, 5th edn, Churchill Livingstone, Edinburgh, 1993.

Part II

The written exams

Chapter 3

Multiple choice question technique (MCQs)

David Protheroe and Chris Williams

The multiple choice question (MCQ) paper is more structured than any other part of the exam, and often aims to test the candidate on the finer detail of the subject. You will need to have detailed knowledge in order to pass. This chapter aims to help you develop your own effective MCQ technique in order to increase your score.

WHAT SHOULD I LEARN?

Obtain and read the Royal College guidelines about the content of the exam.[1] What the guidelines do not tell you is that certain areas of the exam are stressed to a greater extent than others. The following summarises our experience after talking to many candidates over recent years.

PART I MCQ CONTENTS

Fifty questions answered in 90 minutes:

- About 50% is psychopathology.

- The rest is based on the following (in approximate order of priority):

  - Psychodynamic psychotherapy and basic behavioural psychology.

  - Other clinical topics, including physical treatments (such as drugs).

  - Neuroanatomy/neurophysiology/neuro-chemistry.

  - The electroencephalogram (EEG).

PART II MCQ CONTENTS

- **Basic sciences**: 50 questions in 90 minutes. This paper is often felt to be very difficult. There is a large emphasis on psychology, sociology and statistics. You must make sure you know these areas very well.

- **Clinical**: 50 questions in 90 minutes. Be prepared for it. There may be a substantial number of questions on various subspecialities.

PREPARING FOR THE MCQ EXAM

- Practise MCQ questions. A large variety of MCQ books are available. Some of these are better (and more accurate) than others. Of most value are those books which explain the answers so that you add to your knowledge.

- Make your revision more interesting by using MCQs. Some people find that when they continually revise a set of notes over a period of weeks they cease to take any new information in. One way of preventing this is to practise MCQs on each topic shortly after you have revised it. You can then re-read the topic looking for the answers to the questions that you got wrong. This helps highlight particular areas of a subject as important, and allows you to add important details to your notes.

It can be very tempting for candidates approaching the Part II exam to "put off" revising psychology/sociology and statistics. Try to avoid making the mistake of leaving these three topics until just before the exam. These areas are large and need to be learned well. **It is not possible to revise them in only 1 or 2 days**.

TESTING YOUR "FEELING OF KNOWING"

Some people seem to be naturally better at answering MCQs than others. An important factor is the "feeling of knowing" that candidates experience when they read certain questions. You will find that you:

- Know the answer with a high degree of certainty.
- Definitely know that you don't know the answer.
- Have a "feeling of knowing" that the answer is correct, but are not quite sure.

The accuracy of people's "feeling of knowing" varies. Even allowing for negative marking, most people will finish up with a net positive mark if they act in response to their "gut" feelings concerning the "right" answer. It is important to know if this general statistical finding is true for you. It is our experience that approximately one in eight candidates are not able to helpfully trust their "feeling of knowing". For whatever reason, if they trust their "gut" feeling, they will be more often wrong than right. **You need to know if you are one of these people**.

To find this out, do several MCQ papers covering a range of topics. As you do each paper, make your answers using either a black or a red pen:

> • If you know the answer, mark it in **black**.
>
> • If you don't know the answer, leave it **blank**.
>
> • If you have a "feeling of knowing" mark it in **red**.

Now go through the papers and mark them in order to compare your mark when you were certain, and what additional score you would obtain when you use your "feeling of knowing". Try this on a number of papers. If you find that on average you have a net gain of marks by using your instincts, keep doing it! If not, then be cautious about answering questions which you are not at least reasonably sure about.

Incidentally, if your "certain" answers are wrong, you may be overconfident about your knowledge and need to do more factual revision.

MCQ TECHNIQUE

Timing and practical issues

Make sure that you know how the exam is structured. In both Part I and Part II of the exam, 50 questions must be done on each paper in 90 minutes. This means that there are 1.8 minutes per question available.

- You must maintain momentum.

- Read the stem **very** carefully, and all the parts. **Have you understood the question**?

- Do not automatically assume that the examiners are trying to trick you. Avoid agonising over possible hidden meanings, as this is more likely to hinder rather than help your decisions.

- Make sure you put each answer **straight away** on to the right line of the marking sheet. Review this every few questions. It is easy to get your answers out of order. This will cause panic and could cost you the exam. Avoid it!

- Review your progress. You should be aiming to finish every 10 questions in approximately 15 minutes. This allows you time at the end to review your answers.

- If you don't know the correct answer, leave it and come back to the question at the end.

- The "correct" answer to a question is the **generally accepted version of the truth**. If you have some special knowledge of a topic which is at variance with the most prevalent view-point, swallow your pride and save it for the essay question!

The wording of the question

Clues can sometimes be given by the way the questions are asked:

- "Always" and "never" are usually false because it is rare that X never occurs with Y.

- "May" questions are often true. One useful technique that can clarify your thinking here is to reverse the question so that it reads "X may not occur in Y". Try this with some questions in any MCQ book to illustrate to yourself how helpful this technique is.

- "Majority" means at least 50%.

- "Invariably" means 98–99% of the time.

- "Usually" means more than 50%.

- "Frequently" and "often" are poor words to use in MCQs, but mean that something occurs regularly.

- "Rarely", "unusual", "uncommon", "infrequently", and "occasionally" mean less than 5% of the time.

- "A specific feature" means pathognomonic, i.e. occurs in this disease and **no other**.

- "Is associated with" means more commonly than a chance association.

- "Is common in" is another poor stem, but means more than 50%.

Three particularly common stems:

- "A **characteristic** feature" means that it is of diagnostic significance. Its absence might make one doubt the diagnosis.

> - "A **typical** feature" is one which you would expect to be present. It is similar to a characteristic feature.
>
> - "A **recognised** feature" is one that, although it may not characterise a disease, **has been reported**.

EXAMPLE MCQs

The purpose of using examples here is to show that you can gain marks on some questions by using a little knowledge and a lot of technique. General medical questions have been deliberately used rather than psychiatric ones to illustrate the importance of good exam technique. One of us (D.P.) answered the three questions and the subsequent comments reflect the deliberations that he considered in deciding how to respond.

1. Brucellosis:

		My answer
(a)	Cannot be naturally contracted in the UK	F
(b)	May be contracted by drinking untreated milk	T
(c)	Infection may persist for longer than 6 months	T
(d)	Is a cause of depression	DK
(e)	Is characterised by a relative lymphocytosis	DK

I know three things about brucellosis. It is an infection, it is something to do with cows, and I do not think it is a tropical disease. Using this knowledge:

> - Part **(a)** is likely to be false because it seems unlikely that it is impossible to contract a non-tropical disease in the UK.

- Part **(b)** is likely to be true because if you turn the question around thus "It is impossible to contract brucellosis by drinking untreated milk"; my belief that brucellosis is connected with cows means **(b)** is probably true.

- Similarly, if you turn part **(c)** around to become "It is impossible for brucellosis infection to last longer than 6 months", the degree of certainty required in making this statement suggests that the original statement is likely to be true.

- In parts **(d)** and **(e)** the statements clearly go beyond my knowledge and there are no clues in the wording. In this case you are probably better off leaving them. In this case the first three answers are correct so I have scored 60% on a subject about which I know little.

2.   In mumps infection in children:

My answer

(a) Serum amylase may be raised   T
(b) Lymphocytic meningitis is a characteristic
      feature   F
(c) Purulent discharge from the parotid gland
      commonly occurs   F
(d) It is advisable to do viral cultures to confirm
      the diagnosis   F
(e) Abdominal discomfort indicates pancreatic
      involvement   F

I know five things about mumps. It is a common viral infection of the parotid gland and GPs prescribe Calpol to children when they get it. Using what I know:

- Part (a) is likely to be true because the parotid and pancreas are both exocrine glands and to state the reverse of the statement, i.e. "serum amylase can never be raised", seems unlikely. In addition, because part (e) mentions the pancreas again, this makes it more likely that the pancreas is involved.

- Part (b) must be false because surely most kids do not get meningitis when they get mumps.

- Part (c) is false because it is bacterial infections which cause purulent discharges.

- GPs rarely do viral cultures for anything, so (d) must be false. Most children with a fever get tummy ache so its onset with mumps is not likely to herald pancreatic involvement.

3. Hypercholesterolaemia:

My answer

(a) Is usually caused by an enzyme deficiency	F
(b) May present with arthritis	T
(c) Of severe degree is inherited as a dominant trait	T
(d) Is reversed by administration of bile salts	F
(e) Is a characteristic feature of primary biliary cirrhosis	DK

Again with a little knowledge it is possible to score some marks on this question:

- In part (a) the word "usually" gives a clue. "Usually" means more than 50%, and given that I am aware that diet is a very important factor in causing hypercholesterolaemia this seems likely to be false.

- In part **(b)** I would guess "true" purely because of the presence of the word "may". I know that there are inherited disorders of cholesterol metabolism and the presence of a qualifying statement such as "of a severe degree" suggests a true statement in **(c)**.

- The word "reversed" in **(d)** is a very strong claim. Considering that our duodenum already contains significant amounts of bile salts, it is unlikely that a bit more will reverse the problem.

- Part **(e)** is beyond my knowledge and I cannot see any clues in the question so I would answer "Don't know". 80% is a very good mark for a subject I am unfamiliar with!

Using these techniques may help you gain some further marks. It is important to remember that virtually none of the current MCQ books on the market seem to be as hard as the Part II MCQ papers. If you feel that you have done badly on any one paper, **don't panic**! Particularly on the Part II Basic Sciences paper **it is normal to feel you have done badly**. Remember that the overall MCQ mark looks at how you have done compared with everyone else, and that if you have found the paper very hard, it is likely that everyone else will have as well.

SUMMARY

- Practise using a variety of MCQ books.

- Test whether you can trust your "feeling of knowing".

- **Don't panic**: the exam paper often seems very hard.

- Read the questions carefully, looking for clues in the wording.

- Keep checking your answers are on the right place on the answer sheet.

- Maintain momentum.

REFERENCES

[1] *General Information and Regulations for the MRCPsych Examinations.*

This can be obtained from:

The Royal College of Psychiatrists
17 Belgrave Square
London
SW1X 8PG

Tel: 0171 235 2351

Chapter 4

The short answer question paper

Peter Trigwell

Since the current MRCPsych Part II examination was introduced in 1988 it has contained a short answer question (SAQ) paper. The SAQ paper consists of 20 questions and candidates are allowed **one and a half hours** to complete it. Originally this paper consisted of questions which allowed for a variety of answering styles. The questions were something akin to "mini essays", although answers were expected to be brief and lists were allowed where appropriate.

In more recent years the SAQs have tended to be much more **clearly structured**. Most of the questions will ask for a specific number of facts, with the answer sheet having the appropriate number of lines for the answers to be written on.

The College guidelines[1] state that "the Short Answer Question Paper is aimed at testing the accuracy and clarity of the candidate's knowledge. As long as your answer is set out legibly and coherently, there is no reason why it should be written in complete sentences. Listing and the use of a telegrammatic style are acceptable: the space for answers has been structured to help candidates adopt this approach."

Despite the examiners "helping" the candidates in this way there are several points of technique which are essential when sitting this part of the MRCPsych examination. Many candidates expect this part of the exam to be a straightforward regurgitation of factual knowledge in the form of a list. They are surprised how difficult it is to complete the questions fully, even when the question is about a topic which they feel very familiar with.

GENERAL POINTS TO CONSIDER

- Legibility is essential. Each examiner will be marking many papers; they will not be happy with any paper which includes illegible answers needing to be deciphered. The possible result is a very low mark which does not reflect the candidate's true level of knowledge, or the amount of effort they have put in when preparing for the exam. The College guidelines[1] specifically mention the need for answers to be "set out legibly and coherently". You **must** pay attention to this.

- Some abbreviations are so universally used that they are acceptable as part of SAQ answers. 5-HT, GABA, and MAOI are possible examples of this type but if in any doubt at all it is worth writing out all of the abbreviations in long-hand. Other, less universal abbreviations are **not** safe to use.

- The examiner does not make a decision as to whether each of the 20 questions is passed or failed. You can pick up marks from any and all parts of each question; these are then simply added up to decide whether or not you pass the SAQ paper overall.

- A thorough factual knowledge of psychiatry is necessary but not sufficient. Technique is essential in order to do well in the SAQ paper, as in every other part of the MRCPsych exam.

IMPORTANT POINTS OF SAQ TECHNIQUE

Time awareness

Of all the written papers in the MRCPsych Part II exam this is possibly the most difficult to complete fully in the time given. Many candidates who have not practised SAQs in advance, under exam conditions, are surprised at how quickly the time goes on the day of the exam.

- It is essential to arrive in plenty of time for this paper, which tends to be the first paper on the day of the written examinations.

- There are 20 questions to answer in 90 minutes. This allows approximately **4.5 minutes to answer each question**.

- Make a prompt start. If the first one or two questions appear particularly tricky you should move on to later questions and come back to the first ones later.

- You must be constantly aware of the time. Make a point of stopping after you have completed approximately four questions in order to see how the time is going and if you are sticking to the 4.5 minutes allowed for each question.

- If certain questions are easy for you do not spend too long on them. There may be a temptation to put in too much information. A straightforward answer will probably get you the marks; you should press on as you will find the extra time valuable when grappling with the more difficult questions.

Calm approach

A few of the SAQs will seem especially difficult. You may find that you are not sure what the question is asking for and so do not feel able to proceed with **any** of that question. **Do not panic**. It is almost certainly the case that 90% of the candidates in the room with you are feeling the same way about it. Move on and return to that question later. Try to allow time to do so as the answer may suddenly become clearer later on.

Basically, remember that any question which seems very hard for you is probably very hard for everyone.

Breaking answers down into specific points

Many of the questions ask for a list of facts about, or features of, a condition. The problem is often the **size** of the required list rather than any lack of familiarity with the condition on the part of the candidate.

Example

*"List **ten** clinical manifestations of the frontal lobe syndrome."*

Four or five seems reasonable, but **ten**?! This is where breaking down your answers into individual and specific points is so important. **Avoid writing an answer which actually represents a group of points**, when specifying each one of that group of points will earn you a mark for each.

An answer using the "grouping"/non-specific approach might be:

- Behaviour changes.
- Personality changes.
- Mood changes.
- Evidence of cognitive impairment.

The above scores a maximum of 4 out of the possible 10.

An equivalent answer broken down into the specific points could include:

- Disinhibition.

- Facetiousness.

- Loss of initiative.

- Inattention/distractibility.

- Accentuation or obliteration of previous person-ality traits.

- Euphoria.

- Apathy.

- Impaired planning/sequencing of actions.

- Perseveration.

- Slowed thought and motor activity.

- Ataxia.

- Broca's non-fluent dysphasia.

etc.

A selection of 10 such responses gives maximum marks.

The non-specific approach above may well have covered all these points with umbrella terms, such as "personality changes", but specific points earn the marks you need. Viewed in this way it would be reasonably easy to get all the 10 marks available.

Example

"Give 6 indications for ECT."

A non-specific answer might be:

- Depression.
- Certain types of schizophrenia.
- Intractable mania.

This gives 3 marks only.
The preferable, specific approach could include:

- Psychotic/delusional depression.
- Retarded depression/depressive stupor.
- Depression with reduced food/fluid intake.
- Severe depression with high risk of suicide.
- Depression resistant to antidepressant medication.
- Depression in patients unable to tolerate side-effects of antidepressant medication.
- Especially effective in elderly/puerperium.
- Schizophrenic stupor or excitement.
- Severe schizoaffective psychosis.
- Intractable manic states.

etc.

Broad/divergent thinking

Another reason why candidates grind to a premature halt is the use of **narrow thinking**. Any particular question is likely to produce a few instant and, to the candidate, obvious answers. After writing them down, however, there may not appear to be any other answers and full marks will not be gained. It is very important to forget the view *"that's all I seem to be able to think of"* and, instead, take the view *"if they're asking for ten points then I know ten points".* The way to get access to the remaining answers is to make a conscious effort to **broaden your thinking**.

The way to broaden your thinking is to consider what area of your knowledge of psychiatry you are actually using to answer the question. You may be able to add to your answer by switching to other areas. For example, you may be approaching it from the point of view of general adult psychiatry when a switch to thinking of child and adolescent psychiatry, or psychiatry of the elderly, or rehabilitation, liaison psychiatry, or addiction, etc., would stimulate further answers, for further marks.

Example

"List 8 atypical ways in which a depressive episode may present."

Narrow thinking, from the general adult psychiatry perspective, may produce the answer:

- Generalised anxiety symptoms.
- Panic attacks.
- Phobic symptoms.
- Obsessional symptoms.

This gives 4 marks.

Consciously broadening your approach to include other subspeciality areas could generate:

- Somatisation, such as chronic pain or fatigue symptoms.
- Substance misuse.

- Secondary enuresis in a child.

- An apparent dementing process, especially in the elderly.

- Unexplained self-harm or other disturbed behaviour in a patient with mental handicap.

etc.

A similar technique is to think of the headings of the "surgical sieve", as learnt at medical school, in order to stimulate more answers. This is particularly useful in questions about **aetiology**. Some typical headings used are:

- Genetic.

- Traumatic.

- Infective.

- Metabolic.

- Endocrine.

- Vascular.

- Toxic.

- Nutritional.

- Malignant.

- Degenerative.

etc.

Splitting conditions into **primary** and **secondary** may help in a similar way, as may considering the "physical/psychological/ social" triad.

It may be that a switch to your general medical knowledge, or a return to first principles, would help when at first the question seems obscure.

Example

"List 6 appropriate physical investigations for a patient with hyper-cortisolaemia."

This is not the sort of question expected by most candidates in the MRCPsych exam, but it has recently been known for such questions to appear. From a return to first principles, and use of a distant knowledge of such things as excess cortisol production from adrenal tumours and lung carcinomas, and the action of the hypothalamic–pituitary–adrenal axis, many responses can be generated, as follows:

- Serum cortisol estimation.
- Serum ACTH (adrenocorticotrophic hormone).
- Serum corticotrophin releasing factor (CRF).
- Skull radiograph.
- Head computed tomography (CT) or NMR scan.
- Abdominal ultrasound scan.
- Plain chest radiograph.
- Plus thyroid function tests, liver function tests, growth hormone level, prolactin level, etc.

Take note of the marking system

Since the answer paper has been arranged in a way which facilitates list answers, and because the number of marks per answer are specified on the question paper, clues are available as to what the examiners are looking for. Sometimes a list will be requested but with no mention of how many points should be included in it.

Example

"Describe the anatomical pathway taken by cerebrospinal fluid in the central nervous system."
(10 marks)

....
....
....
....
....
....
....
....
....
....

The fact that 10 marks are available (and 10 lines are provided) helps in structuring your answer. Hence:

- Choroid plexus.

- Lateral ventricles.

- Interventricular foraminae (of Monro).

- Third ventricle.

- Cerebral aqueduct (of Sylvius).

- Fourth ventricle.

- Median foramen (of Magendie).

- Lateral foraminae (of Luschka).

- Subarachnoid space.

- Arachnoid villi/superior sagittal sinus/venous blood stream.

The above is highly likely to gain maximum marks.

Example

"Describe the 'Hamilton cuff method' for determining that a seizure has occurred in electroconvulsive therapy."
(3 marks total)

In this example you can be fairly confident that points will be awarded for:

- Sphygmomanometer cuff inflated to **above systolic** blood pressure.
- Done **before relaxant** given.
- Observe effects of seizure on isolated limb.

(It is perfectly acceptable to underline important parts of the answer if you wish.)

Understand/answer the question as asked on the paper

Mistakes can be made, and valuable marks lost, in the SAQ paper by reading the question quickly and not being careful to answer what is actually asked. This is obviously the case also in the other (essay and MCQ) written papers.

Example

*"List **ten** side-effects of antipsychotic drugs, including at least three autonomic and three extrapyramidal effects."*

In this case it is essential to satisfy the examiners by supplying three of each specified type of side-effect first, then completing the rest of the answer, e.g.:

- Dry mouth.

- Blurred vision.

- Urinary retention.

- Bradykinesia.

- Rigidity.

- Tremor.

- Constipation.

- Galactorrhoea.

- Sialorrhoea.

- Hypothermia.

Example:

"Give the incidence rate per 1000 births of:

Maternity blues
Postnatal depression
Puerperal psychosis."

Most candidates know the incidence rates of these conditions, but they may be used to expressing them as percentages. The answers given would, therefore, be:

- 50.

- 10.

- 0.1–0.2.

This would gain **no marks whatsoever** as the question specifies the units to be used, so that the correct and only acceptable answers are:

- 500.
- 100 (80–140 would probably be accepted).
- 1 to 2.

Number of points requested

It is very important to take note of **how many points are required** in a list-type answer. In some of the examples above, many more than the required number of responses are listed. This would **not** be advisable in the examination itself.

The examiner will have a list of acceptable answers to help him or her judge when marking the paper, but if you write down 10 points when only 5 are asked for **the first 5 and only those answers will be marked**. (This will remain the case even if the first 5 happen to be incorrect and the last 5 correct!)

As a result, it is essential to write down those answers you are most confident of first, up to the number required.

No negative marking

Unlike the MCQ paper, there is no "negative marking" in the SAQ paper. This means that you should **attempt every question**.

Towards the end of the SAQ exam you should **go through it again, looking for gaps** where you have not yet written an answer. Even if you think that the only answer you can think of is extremely unlikely you must "have a go" and fill the gaps with possibilities.

You could be lucky and gain an extra mark or two, and you will certainly not be penalised in any way – no matter how ridiculous the answer may actually be.

Sources of information and revision

Although larger texts and other literature need to be studied, there are some small revision books for the MRCPsych which are set out in a similar way to SAQ answers. These are well worth reading and are useful preparation for the SAQ part of the MRCPsych Part II examination. For example, many candidates have found the following two texts particularly useful in this way:

- *Examination Notes in Psychiatry*[2].

- *Examination Notes on the Scientific Basis of Psychiatry*[3].

Common questions

Certain topics lend themselves very well to SAQ type questions, especially in list form. This means that **certain questions come up time and time again**. You should try to spot such areas and commit them to memory, so that they can be easily and reliably reproduced on the day of the exam.

Such standard/classic facts will be asked for in total, the examiners wanting, for example, **all 12** of the "Curative factors" in group therapies according to Yalom[4].

The following is a list of other such important areas. You may be able to add to it.

- Names, basic features and age ranges of Piaget's four stages of childhood cognitive development.

- Features of attachment behaviour in human infants.

- Risk factors for the development of tardive dyskinesia.

- Beck's "cognitive triad", and errors of intellectual processing.

- Stages of molecular genetic techniques, e.g. Southern blotting and RFLPs (restriction fragment length polymorphisms).

- Negative symptoms of schizophrenia.

- Prognostic indicators in schizophrenia.

- Features of temporal lobe epilepsy.

- Points of note in assessing suicidal intent/risk following an episode of deliberate self-harm.

- Features of a normal distribution curve.

- Certain definitions (e.g. impairment, disability, handicap).

- Metabolites of serotonin, dopamine and noradrenaline.

- Enzymes involved in these metabolites' formation.

- Amino acids which act as neurotransmitters in the brain.

- Proteins which act as neurotransmitters in the brain.

- Major sites of dopamine neurones in the brain, and their projections.

You may think you know these answers – try writing them down now. It could be worth another look!

SUMMARY

- Time awareness is essential.
- A calm approach is needed.
- Break answers down into specific points.
- Use broad/divergent thinking.
- Take note of the marking system.
- Understand/answer the question as asked.
- Note the number of points requested.
- No negative marking (answer **all** the questions).
- **Practise SAQs**, especially common questions/lists.

REFERENCES

[1] Chief Examiner, *MRCPsych Part II Examination. Short Answer Question Paper – Guidance to Candidates*, The Royal College of Psychiatrists, London, 1990.
[2] J. Bird and G. Harrison, *Examination Notes in Psychiatry*, 2nd edn, Wright, Bristol, 1987.
[3] T.G. Dinan, *Examination Notes on the Scientific Basis of Psychiatry*, Wright, Bristol, 1985.
[4] I.D. Yalom, *The Theory and Practice of Group Psychotherapy*, 3rd edn, Basic Books, New York, 1985.

Chapter 5

Essay technique

David Yeomans

When did you last write an essay? If like many exam candidates you have not written an essay for years, this chapter should revive forgotten skills and provide you with some techniques for exam success.

The essay is not negatively marked, but you still need to demonstrate a factual and accurate understanding of the question. Furthermore, you must present that account in good English using correct spelling and grammar. Your essay needs a structure and will benefit from a lively writing style. Your examiner, after marking several essays which are meandering and tedious, may well be tired and irritable. Cheer them up with a legible and interesting piece of prose!

PREPARATION

When you draw up your revision timetable be sure to set aside regular time to practise essays. Writing is physically tiring and is a skill which you may not have practised for several years. By the end of your revision you should have written 10–20 essay plans and at least two full-length pieces.

Reading is your major source of factual information. Textbooks plus revision books will give you enough factual material to pass, but additional material from specialist books, journals, clinical experience and conferences will increase your chances. You cannot read everything, so be selective. Review articles in major journals (e.g. *British Journal of Psychiatry*) and review journals (e.g. *Current Opinion*) are useful. Read the exam syllabus in the Inceptor's Handbook (from the Royal College of Psychiatrists) to see which areas you need to know and which you don't. Send off for past papers and obtain the most recent exam papers from colleagues who have recently taken the exam.

ESSAY SPOTTING

There are several assumptions underlying the technique of essay spotting:

* Certain topics are important and these tend to be repeated.

* If such a topic has not come up recently then the chances of it appearing as a question in the next exam (your exam) are increased.

* Currently topical issues are often set on the essay paper (e.g. nationwide changes in service provision, Mental Health Act, prominent review articles). Look at the editorials and reviews which have appeared in the last 12 months of the *Psychiatric Bulletin* and the *British Journal of Psychiatry*.

Work out what major topics you wish to cover. Many candidates find it useful to produce a collection of "essay plans". If you prepare 15 to 20 topics, at least some of them can be included in whole or part form in the actual exam.

STRUCTURE

What is an essay? It is a long written piece held together by a **structure** and contains **arguments** supported by **information**. A common structure for an essay is an *introduction*, then the *arguments*, followed by your *conclusion*. This may need to be modified depending on how the essay question is asked. A very open question such as "Describe the uses of medical audit" requires you to define the structure yourself. A question such as *"Discuss the effects of antidepressants on the course and outcome of anxiety disorders"* is more clearly defined, but you must still impose some structure to your answer. Your answer can be structured using the following techniques:

- **Six useful questions** are: *"Who? What? Why? Where? When? How?"* When tackling the essay ask yourself these questions to help produce a critical discussion. Think about what terms the question uses. *What* is medical audit? *Who* is interested in audit? *Why* should doctors get involved? *How* is anxiety defined? *How many* different antidepressants are there? *What* is outcome? *How* is it measured?

- **Helicoptering** (Fig. 5.1). A helicopter can hover miles up in the sky to obtain a broad view of the situation. It can descend to various points in that landscape to see more detail. You can do this in an essay by focusing in and out to offer both a general overview and also specific detail and argument.

- **Expansion**. Before setting pen to paper expand the question to its limits by considering all the subject areas you can include. Helpful

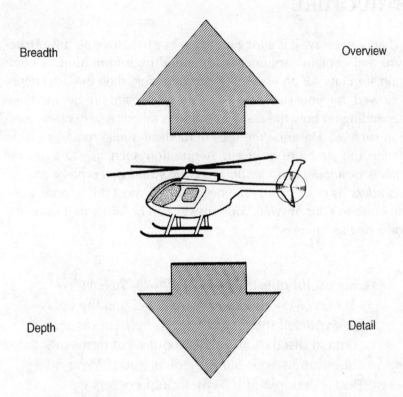

Fig. 5.1. Helicoptering.

subheadings to expand the scope of your thinking (and hence your essay) include:

– Biological, psychological and social aspects.

– Acute, intermediate and long term.

– Male and female differences.

– Age differences.

– Cultural differences.

– "Non-medical" factors such as the impact on carers, media influences (the author

> managed to quote a daytime TV chat show in the essay), politics, and finance.
>
> – Past, present and future implications.

WORKED EXAMPLES

Example 1

Candidates on the Leeds Examination Technique Course were asked to use the above techniques to create **essay plans**. Although no one felt prepared for the task, one group produced the following essay structure within 10 minutes:

Question

"Discuss medical classification and how it has been applied in psychiatry."

Answer

- **Introduction** (*why is classification necessary?*):
  - Communication.
  - Universal use.
  - Predict prognosis.
  - It aids research so that different researchers can study similar patients.
  - Implications for treatment.
- **Classification methods**:
  - Syndromal (grouping of symptoms and signs).

- Aetiology (infective, trauma, genetic, etc.).

- Course (acute, chronic or remitting).

- Outcome.

- Multiaxial definitions (or a combined biopsychosocial model).

- **Application of classification models in psychiatry**:

  - The current systems: ICD, DSM.

  - Lack of success, lack of clear aetiologies and the limitations of syndromal classification.

  - Outcome prediction actually quite poor.

  - Historical perspective, e.g. Kraepelin.

- **Conclusions**:

  - Slow but steady progress is being made.

  - More consensus than before.

  - Future hope to include more aetiological and pathological data with multi-axial descriptions taken into account.

This essay structure demonstrates some of the techniques described above. First of all, you **must read the question in full**. A simple approach with an **introduction**, **arguments**, and **conclusion** is used. There is a clear structure. The candidates in this case **defined what** classification is and **why** it is used. They **helicoptered** down from the two broad questions on classification and application and split each up into several headings. For some of the headings they helicoptered down further to give detailed examples which illustrate the benefits and pitfalls of using diagnostic systems. They then helicoptered up again to allow a wider discussion of the arguments. The essay structure is **critical** and asks **how** successful classification is in psychiatry. It looks to **what** the future may hold and **expands** the question a little beyond what was asked. Perhaps it could have included some consideration of **cultural differences** and similarities. You may already have different ideas of how you would answer this question. Why not try them out now?

Example 2

Question

"How can exploratory psychotherapy lead to a worsening of a patient's condition? What can be done to reduce this?"

Answer

- **Introduction**:
  - *Exploratory psychotherapy*: dynamic psychotherapy, types/methods; individual/group/family; in children and adults.
  - *Worsening*:
    - (i) In therapy – transference/countertransference issues, and risks of dependency.
    - (ii) Out of therapy – acting out; also to consider problems in work or with their family.
    - (iii) General – risks of parasuicide/self-harm, anxiety or depression.
- **Arguments**: this went on to discuss the above

ideas, and particularly to discuss the "worsening" in terms of overall outcome.

- **What can be done to reduce worsening?**:

  - Patient selection, including liaison with referrers.

  - Training and supervision of psychotherapists.

  - Conjoint work and treatment (e.g. additional medication from GPs).

  - The importance of clear communication and continuity of treatment.

  - Monitor the mental state closely.

  - Assess defence mechanisms for potential vulnerability to psychological treatment approaches.

  - Pay attention to transference and counter-transference issues and difficulties.

  - Give adequate preparation for times of absence by the therapist.

  - Consider the frequency of sessions and the risks of dependency occurring.

The candidates' reaction to this essay title was interesting. Initially they felt great pessimism when given this question to attempt. They said that they would never have chosen this topic in an exam, and felt that they would answer it very badly because they did not have any specialised expertise in this field. None expected to produce such an extensive outline until they applied the techniques taught above. They were surprised to find out exactly how much they really knew. Had this been the only question they could remotely hope to answer, this technique-based approach would have given them more than a fighting chance of passing.

THE ROLE OF THE EXAMINER

Pity the examiner who has to mark a lot of essays on the same question. Remember he or she may well be bored and miserable, sat at home perhaps, with dogs barking and kids crying. It is your task to present them with a clearly legible, well-written, structured essay which stands out from all the others.

WHAT TO DO

Write legibly. **I know of an examiner who failed a candidate in 5 seconds because the essay was unreadable**. Consider writing double spaced. This makes your essay easier on the eye and simpler to mark. Break up the text with headings, lists, diagrams and tables, where appropriate. (Take a look at your textbooks and see how they present information. Each chapter in the book is itself an essay.) Use colour (e.g. a red pen) to highlight important points, or subheadings using underlining.

When you sit the essay paper, spend a few minutes before you start writing to prepare an **essay plan**. Write out your essay structure at the beginning of the essay and label it as the "essay outline." You can then refer back to it as you write in order to maintain the structure and keep track of the remaining time. Cross out those areas you have covered so that you can see how the essay is progressing. Take time to review the content intermittently in case any fresh ideas come to mind.

Write naturally, but consider the following. Short sentences add impact. Long sentences with no punctuation such as commas that go on for line after line and talk about different subjects without so much as a pause between them do tend to confuse and the examiner does not want to re-read the essay 10 times to work out what you are trying to say. See?

Show the examiners that you can order information, and

make the presentation and structure clear by the use of subheadings.

• Bullet points can be very effective in lists.

References need not be given in full. Names will usually suffice.

WHAT NOT TO DO

Don't make things up. Don't waffle about irrelevances. Do not write about a totally different question just because you have prepared an essay plan about it. You will get no marks unless you answer the question which is asked. Remember this point when you have spotted a question. You need to tailor the prepared answer to the question on the exam paper. Do not be unbalanced in your arguments. Remember that your essay reveals things about you. Examiners may be concerned if, for example, you appear to have no consideration for patients' well-being . Finally, remember that an essay requires a reasonably lengthy piece of writing – one page is not enough!

WHAT ARE YOUR BLINDSPOTS?

When you write a practice essay, ask someone to comment on it critically. You may be unaware of habitual spelling or grammatical errors. You may not notice a tendency to leave words unfinished (the author has this proble). Let someone else discover your blindspots, but be critical of their criticism. In the end you have to rely on your own style.

SUMMARY

• Practise writing full length essays.

• Prepare 10–20 outline essay plans using spotting techniques.

- Read the questions carefully. Tailor prepared essay plan to the exam question.

- Create an essay structure using critical questions, helicoptering and expansion techniques.

- Write legibly.
- Make your essay interesting.

Part III

The clinical exam

Chapter 6

Preparing for the long case

Chris Williams

Many people sit the MRCPsych exams, yet only approximately 45% of candidates pass each time. To pass the exam as a whole, you **must** be successful in the clinical exam. **How can you stand out as being someone who should pass**? The general principles of doing well in the clinical exams are to organise your knowledge, making what you say:

- Clear.
- Relevant.
- Interesting.

Remember:

- You have done this all before.
- It is not a test of academic knowledge; this is covered in the written papers.
- Clear communicators consistently do well.

- **You are presenting yourself** not merely the case.

- You are also being asked to demonstrate your skills as a clinician.

The examiner's key question is **"Would I trust this person to be my Senior Registrar when I am away on holiday**?" You therefore need to convey an impression of reliability and safety. In the same way that in a driving test you need to make the instructor feel safe while you drive, in the case of sitting the exams you need to show the examiners that you are a safe, sensible and competent clinician who could be trusted to look after their patients.

PREPARATION

The good news is that you know in advance what areas the examiners are interested in. You will be asked to present your case summary, including the mental state examination, present and justify your differential diagnosis and, in the case of the Part II exam, go on to discuss possible management plans. To prepare for this:

- Know what is expected of you. Read the Royal College guidelines concerning the exam; these tell you about the content and structure of the exam.

- Practise presenting cases.

- Take opportunities to present cases (ward rounds, clinic, etc.).

- For some of the cases, make sure that you are asked to interview the patient in front of the mock examiner. This is something which is rarely practised, but is important.

- Seek supervised training in interviewing skills. **Watch yourself presenting on video**. This is the most effective way of changing! It has the added advantage that the actual exam will be no more stressful than this.

- Practise presenting to peers, and also watch them presenting. Attempt to mark each other's performance using the mark sheet (shown on page 64). You will gain from seeing how others present their cases, and they will also learn from you.

MOCK CLINICAL EXAMS

Make sure that you do mock clinical exams on each of the main areas of psychiatry. These are common problems seen in psychiatric practice, and hence are common in exams:

- Depressive disorder.
- Schizophrenia.
- Anxiety disorders.
- Obsessive compulsive disorder.
- Alcohol abuse/dependence.
- Eating disorders.

Also do mock exams with a variety of **different examiners** who have different theoretical and clinical backgrounds. If there are any College examiners at the hospital where you work, it would be well worth arranging to carry out at least one exam with them as well. Be willing to accept their feedback and suggestions to change. Ultimately, however, you are seeking to develop a clinical interview and presentation style with which **you** are happy.

When you do the practice exams, try to obtain **specific feedback**. This will help you identify your relatively stronger and weaker areas. An assessment sheet such as the one below may aid this and can be used by others (for example your peers in a study group) to rate your performance. You can also use it yourself if you are analysing your presentation on videotape.

Mock clinical exam assessment sheet

Examiner: **Candidate:**

Initial case presentations:
The ability to pick out the salient features of the case and present these clearly and coherently is stressed. The organisation of information is particularly important. The assessment of **relevant physical factors** should be recognised in the mark.
(7–10 minutes)

Interviewing the patient:
Politeness and professional attitude. The ability to firmly but politely control the interview without dominating, and at the same time cover the appropriate clinical questions quickly, clearly and efficiently.
(5 minutes)

Discussion of the differential diagnosis, aetiology, management and prognosis of the case:
Paying particular regard to social and psychological treatments as well as purely physical approaches.
(15 minutes)

Overall mark:
A general discussion with the candidate would probably be the most help rather than an overall statement of Pass or Fail.

Comments:
Helpful ways to improve presentation and organisation of material.

PREDICTING AND PRACTISING CASES

Try to remember that the hospital where you sit the examination will tend to have the same types of patient that you see in your own clinical practice. The hospital has to provide approximately 20–30 patients for the exams and these are therefore likely to include both inpatients and outpatients. Think through in advance how you will assess, present and manage each of the following clinical cases. It is not necessary to carry out mock exams on each of these, but you should try to do so, and you should certainly **think each case through thoroughly**. Many find it useful to either write down full assessment and management plans of a "typical" case, or to test and be tested by peers who are also taking the exam.

Write out full assessment and management plans for each of the following:
(Be able to present these concisely and efficiently in an informed manner.)

- Depressive disorder (including psychotic depression).
- Schizophrenia (and drug-induced psychosis).
- Alcohol or substance abuse.
- Anxiety disorders.
- Obsessive–compulsive disorder.
- Agoraphobia or other phobias.
- Hypochondriasis and abnormal illness behaviour.

- Mild/moderate dementia cases (these will be accompanied by an informant).

- Eating disorders.

- Any area that the hospital is known to specialise in.

It is possible that a patient with mental handicap or a child will be used in the exam. If so, they would always be accompanied by an informant.

Do not attempt to visit or contact the clinical staff or wards of the hospital you will be examined at. This can lead to you being disqualified from the exam.

COMING TO THE EXAM

Think:

- What will I wear?

- What impression do I want to give?

- What will I do over the lunchtime break? (Do not smell of drink or smoke.)

How can I arrive on time?

It is surprising how often this causes problems. Expect the unexpected (traffic jams, rail strikes, losing your car keys, etc.). **If you are late for any part of the exam it will leave you feeling tense, pressured and unlikely to perform well**. It can destroy months of hard work, and mean that you will have to repeat all your revision once again. Definitely consider staying overnight in a **nice** hotel (not noisy). It is worth the money. A long drive with an early start can seem too far on the day because you will feel stressed. You will probably not have slept well and being "on-site" can make a big difference. One of the authors went out with another candidate to have a "relaxing" meal on the night before the written exams. Unfortunately he ate so much curry that he was then unable to sleep, and ended up trying to develop bulimic tendencies in the toilet. Beware!

The overriding thing to have in mind is that the patients chosen for the exams will be **appropriate** for the level of exam you are sitting. Sometimes patients seem very complex. You can still pass the exam by keeping calm and concentrating on technique. Chapter 4 will show you a simple, systematic approach to effective clinical assessment and presentation.

EXAMINERS' ADVICE TO CANDIDATES TAKING THE MRCPsych CLINICAL EXAMS

The following section summarises comments that have been distilled from talking to a number of past and present College examiners. They highlight several areas which candidates fall down on time and time again. Their recommendations show how using effective examination techniques could markedly improve your performance.

Organise your presentation:

- Have your notes clearly ordered.
- Ensure good time management so that you are able to present your case summary in less than ✗ 10 minutes (including the differential diagnosis).
- Anticipate questions.
- Have a logical progression through the presentation.
- Do a brief physical examination, and mention it.

Initial presentation:

- Diagnosis in ICD 10 or DSM IV.
- You must be able to discuss this and justify your differential diagnoses.

Interview with the patient:

- Show courtesy and sensitivity, but maintain control of the interview.
- Give a good explanation to the patient of what is happening.
- Structure the interview so that you are able to cover the questions (usually two) which the examiners have specified.

Discussion of the case:

- You must be able to answer *"**Why** has this patient presented at this particular time?"*
- Avoid generalisations, and make your answers **specific** to this particular patient.
- Include physical, psychological and social investigations and treatment.
- Demonstrate a **safe**, considered approach to management. Make the examiners feel that you are reliable and sensible.

Presenting yourself:

- Have sensible and professional dress.
- Show a confident manner.
- Follow and listen to questions carefully.
- Be prepared to reconsider your conclusions in the light of new evidence, where appropriate.

Read the College *Instructions to Candidates*[1] carefully. These are constantly updated, and provide useful guidance on the timing and content of the exams.

REFERENCES

[1] Royal College of Psychiatrists, *Instructions to Candidates*, Royal College of Psychiatrists, 17 Belgrave Square, London SW1X 8PG (Tel. 0171 235 2351).

Chapter 7

The clinical assessment

Chris Williams

WINNING OVER THE PATIENT

- Make sure you arrive on time!

- Introduce yourself to the patient.

- Say that you are nervous too!

- Explain that you need to take notes.

- **Apologise** in advance for having to interrupt them; say why (it is an exam, time pressures, etc.).

- When you do interrupt, say something like *"I'm sorry to interrupt you again, but I need to ask . . . "*.

- Be polite and professional.

- **Don't panic** if it seems a very complex case. The examiners know this and will make allowances.

BE ORGANISED AS YOU TAKE THE HISTORY

Nothing creates an impression of disorganisation more than a flurry of paper during the presentation. This can be reduced by using a few simple techniques:

- **Write on only one side of the paper.**
- Number the sheets.
- Organise your information clearly as you take the history.
- Use clear headings (Personal History, Family History, etc.).
- Consider writing the headings down at the start of the exam. This can help you pace your history taking, and also prevents you forgetting to ask about any central and important areas.

It is not the place here to go through in detail how to take a psychiatric history. This is described in all basic psychiatric text books. A good description is in *The Oxford Textbook of Psychiatry*[1]. We suggest that you read the chapters on the psychiatric history and mental state in detail and repeatedly practise areas such as testing the cognitive state.

While taking the history use a style most examiners will recognise.

For example:

- Presenting complaint/history of presenting complaint (PC/HPC).

- Personal history.

- Premorbid personality (PMP).

- Family history (FH).

- Social – are **any other professionals** or services involved (Day Hospital, Community Psychiatric Nurse, Social Worker, etc.)? Ask about housing problems, **alcohol and substance misuse**. Are they under a **Section** of the Mental Health Act?

- **Forensic history.**

- Past medical history.

- Past psychiatric history (always including post-partum problems and **deliberate self-harm**).

- Drugs/allergies. **Do not forget depots or current ECT.**

- Full mental state examination. (Know how to do **cognitive testing**.)

Always include the presence or absence of suicidal ideas and behaviour.

(**Remember to ask about the topics in bold.** They are the most commonly forgotten.)

- **Maintain momentum**. You cannot afford to run out of time.

- **Leave gaps** between each area on your history sheets. You **will** forget questions and this allows you to fit in later questions without creating an unreadable mass of extra notes scribbled in margins.

- You can always ask the patient what diagnosis they have been given, and also what treatments or investigations they have had. This can offer very useful clues!

- Aim to finish in 45 minutes. Ask the patient to stay.

- Check what you have forgotten/clarify points.

- Consider using a **red pen** to mark important key areas which you will read out in the presentation.

- Thank the patient and mention that you will be asked to interview them again in front of the examiners.

The physical examination scores marks even if brief, e.g.:

- Pulse.

- Blood pressure.

- Evidence of autonomic overarousal (e.g. sweating, pallor, tremor).

- Stigmata of thyroid or liver disease.

- Evidence of previous injury (self-cutting, etc.).

- Anything relevant. If the patient has only one leg or is in a wheelchair, say so.

CLUSTERING QUESTIONS

A very important technique to learn is that of **clustering questions together**. In psychiatry, diagnoses are largely made by observing if particular symptoms aggregate together in patterns that are felt to represent specific disorders or syndromes. Most examiners have a model in their minds of the cluster of symptoms which make up each diagnosis, e.g. "depressive disorder". These clusters have been formalised in the various diagnostic systems such as ICD 10 and DSM IV. How then is this relevant to the exam situation?

Examiners do not know very much information about the patient you have seen. All they know is a basic written summary from the Senior House Officer or Registrar looking after them. What you need to do is to **paint a picture of the patient** for them. In order to present this clearly to the examiners, it is vital to **cluster symptoms together logically while taking the history, and therefore while presenting**. This is key to a good presentation. When, for example, you mention depressed mood the examiners will want to know if the patient fits their own (or the ICD) model of depression. They will therefore expect a description of not only how depressed the mood is, the presence of anhedonia, mood reactivity, etc., but also whether there is any evidence of "biological" symptoms of depression, and to what extent the depression has affected the person's life.

Thus, if you are asking about depression ask about all these areas **at one time** so that your history contains a clear focused summary. Write the symptoms down on one part of the paper so that they are presented (clustered) clearly on your sheets and hence when you present. Don't allow yourself to be distracted by the patient when taking the history. In some cases you may have to come back to clarify things later, but do this all on the same sheet of paper so that everything you have found out about a particular problem area is found together in that one spot. This will help you to give a clear presentation.

Two typical "clusters" of questions covering depression and anxiety are presented below. Each of these have a similar structure. Try to create your own individualised clusters which you will be able to remember easily. Practise these until you can go through them quickly and reliably.

Clustering symptoms of depression

1. **Mood**: Severity/anhedonia/weepiness/reactivity/ hopelessness/loss of confidence/self-esteem/ indecisiveness/suicidal ideas, etc.

2. **Biological symptoms**: Diurnal variation of mood, poor appetite, weight loss, etc.

3. **How it has affected the patient**:

> • "What have you stopped doing since becoming depressed?"
>
> • "How has it affected you, your family and work?"

Clustering symptoms of anxiety

1. **Mood**: How severe is the anxiety? Is it generalised or focused as a phobic state. Does the anxiety ever rise to a peak and cause panic attacks? If so, what are the precipitants of this, and how does the person cope?

2. **Biological symptoms**: Is there evidence of marked somatic anxiety? It can be helpful to cluster the questions by asking about evidence of sympathetic, parasympathetic symptoms, and also for the symptoms caused by hyperventilation.

Sympathetic nervous system:

- Rapid heart.
- Palpitations.
- Muscle tension pains (e.g. chest pain).
- Tremor.
- Sweaty, clammy.
- Flushed or blanched.

Parasympathetic nervous system:

- Nausea.
- Vomiting.
- Loose motions/diarrhoea.
- Frequency of urine.

Hyperventilation:

- Dizzy.
- Blurred vision.
- Depersonalisation/derealisation.
- Sweaty/hot.
- Dry mouth.
- Chest pain.
- Subjective shortness of breath.

3. How it has affected the patient:

Is there any evidence of **avoidance**. This has important implications for treatment.

- "What have you stopped doing since becoming anxious?"
- "How has it affected you, your family and work?"

Create your own **symptom-cluster checklists**, asking about paranoid ideas/schizophrenia, and also assessing the nature of suicidal ideas. Both these are common in exams. You will find that the skills learned in doing this will also be useful for the time when you have to interview the patient in front of the examiners, because it will teach you to be organised, structured and clear.

THE VITAL QUARTER HOUR

Try to complete the basic history in approximately 45 minutes. The critical time which can make or break any clinical presentation is the 15 minutes that you have left from your hour with the patient. **Check through your sheets while the patient is in the room**. There will also be 5–10 minutes **in addition** before you go in to see the examiners after the patient is taken out of the room. **This is the key time to gather your thoughts**.

You do not have time to re-write or indeed read out the entire history for the examiners, therefore **make sure that your notes are organised and structured clearly as you take the history**. Practise this in mock exams. Consider spending some time marking those areas that you are going to read out with a red pen. This will help you focus on the important features of the case.

Remember that the purpose of the history is to try to **understand** the person and their problems. You want to paint a picture for the examiners of the patient you have seen. Focus what you say in order to paint this picture effectively.

STRUCTURING YOUR PRESENTATION

Think in advance about the six areas you will be expected to cover:

1. Presentation of the history and mental state.

2. Differential diagnosis (with justifications).

3. Aetiology. The three Ps:

- Predisposing factors
- Precipitating factors
- Perpetuating factors

4. Investigations (social, psychological, physical).

5. Management (social, psychological, physical).

6. Prognosis (short term, long term).

PREPARING THE HISTORY AND MENTAL STATE

You have approximately 7–10 minutes to present the whole case. Of this, **it is the opening few minutes that matter the most**. It is during this time that you will present either a favourable or unfavourable impression of yourself. Examiners, being human, tend to label you as clearly passing or failing early on in the presentation. In our experience, it is quite difficult to switch between these labels once they have been applied; therefore it is vital to have the "right" label attached as soon as possible. How can you make this happen?

Prepare your opening few sentences. If the patient has been a difficult or poor historian say so now and possibly again later, but only once more. Do not overstate this. Next, **write out the first two or three sentences of your presentation**.

1. **A summary demographic statement.**
   Write this out in advance: one sentence only
   (see example below).

2. **The key problems in the case.**
   Write these out in advance: one or two
   sentences only (see example below).

> - What are the **key problems**?
>
> - You need to **focus** the history on these.
>
> - Can you tell the wood from the trees?
>
> - There **is** time to do this.

3. **Now read out the salient features of the whole history and mental state examination.**

> - State the **headings** whilst presenting the case in order to give clear "**signposts**" of where you are in the presentation ("*Key features from the personal history include: . . .*", etc.).
>
> - Make sure that the flow of the history is **logical**, and present the history in a form which most examiners will recognise (see the discussion on taking the history, above).

- Make sure that you communicate to the examiners that any important screening questions have been asked, even if there is no positive reply. For example *"On direct questioning there was no evidence of any of the first rank symptoms of schizophrenia"*, or
  "There was evidence of early morning wakening, but no other biological symptoms of depression".

Remember:

- Keep calm.
- Modify the following suggested model to fit your cases. If you already have a model that you are happy with, then don't change it much unless you want to.

- Definitely **do not change your regular style of presentation on the day of the exam**. It never works. Get used to one style of presentation, and stick to it.

- Be interested and interesting! Vary your voice tone as you present, and make good eye contact with both examiners.

PRESENTING THE CASE

To illustrate this approach, the following summarises the structure of a typical presentation:

1. **A demographic summary sentence**.

   "The gentleman I saw is Mr S.J., who is a 33-year-old married man who lives with his wife and two children in a council house."

2. **One or two sentences summarising the key problem areas**.
   This is the main focus of the history. **Write this out in advance**.

   *"He has had problems which began after the breakdown of his marriage, and this has left him feeling **depressed**, **anxious** and **suicidal**. This led him to take an **overdose** which precipitated the admission to hospital. There are a number of associated difficulties, including a lack of **social support** and isolation which have aggravated his situation."*

3. **Key parts of the rest of the history and mental state**.

   "He presented two weeks ago with . . . "

   Then on to describe the main complaint (e.g. the "Depressive cluster" of symptoms) and each of the other problem areas one by one.

   - Read these off your sheets.
   - They should not need to be re-written.
   - Go through the rest of the history reading out

the relevant items. **Draw attention to positive findings, and important negatives** (e.g. first rank symptoms, example as before).

- **Use set phrases to save time**.

"Mr S.J. describes a normal birth, development, childhood and schooling history. He left school at sixteen and . . . "

This implies that you have asked about these areas. (Make sure that you have!)

The purpose of the history is to paint a picture of the person, their problems and supports. Mention relevant **p**redisposing, **p**recipitating or **p**erpetuating factors as you go through the history. For example, in a depressed patient you may find:

- Death of mother when he was young.
- No job outside the home.
- Lack of a supportive relationship.
- Three or more children at home below the age of fourteen.[2]

These factors are all now felt to exert their effect via **low self-esteem**; therefore look for other things in the history that would lead to similar problems.

You should not need to write out more than the first three or four sentences of the presentation (i.e. the summary demographic statement and the key presenting problems). After this it is merely a matter of deciding what parts of the rest of the history sheets to read out.

After presenting the salient points of the history and the mental state examination, you will move on to present the differential diagnosis, etc.

THE DIFFERENTIAL DIAGNOSIS

Consider "psychiatric" *and* "physical" differential diagnoses.

- There is often no single right answer.
- *"There are a number of possibilities which include . . . "*
- If it is obvious, state what you feel the diagnosis is.
- Show that you know that patients can change, and that your opinions are not fixed, but based upon the evidence that you find *now* at interview.

If it is very complicated, DON'T PANIC. Instead use a phrase like:

*"This is a very complicated case. After only an hour with the patient and without the chance to review old notes or talk to an informant, I have a **range** of differential diagnoses, but at the present time I would not be able to put them into any definite order. However my differential at present is . . . "*

- If someone appears guarded, consider including paranoid psychosis in the differential diagnosis.

State the diagnosis you favour at the present time. Using information from the history make the case **for and against** each of the differential diagnoses in turn.

Standardised differential diagnoses

You will be required to use the ICD 10 classification in the exams. You should therefore familiarise yourself with this classification. It can be very helpful to have pre-prepared a list of "standardised" differential diagnoses for the common presenting complaints that you come across. These are not lists merely to regurgitate in exams, but instead help you to remember the **range of diagnostic possibilities** (both psychiatric and physical) for you to consider. Having these to fall back on can be a great help if anxiety levels are high and you are finding it difficult to think effectively during the exam. Do remember to only state these if you **really are** considering them in the differential for this particular case.

Differential diagnosis of depression using ICD 10

1. Bipolar affective disorder:

- Specify type of current episode.

2. Depressive episode:

- Mild or moderate depressive episode ± somatic symptoms.
- Severe depressive episode ± psychotic symptoms.

3. Recurrent depressive disorder.

4. Persistent mood disorders.

- Dysthymia.
- Cyclothymia.

5. Adjustment disorder.

6. **Mixed affective episode**.

7. **Organic cause**.

- Hypothyroidism.

- Alcohol dependency.

- Other. **Only state actual possibilities**. Don't just say *"or an organic cause of the disorder"*. You must be specific about what you have in mind, and give evidence to support it, e.g. *"Hypothyroidism, in view of the history of loss of energy and marked weight gain"*.

Differential diagnosis of paranoid ideas using ICD 10

- Schizophrenia.

- Schizotypal disorder.

- Schizoaffective disorder.

- Persistent delusional disorders.

- Acute and transient psychotic disorders.

- Schizoid personality disorder.

- Mania with psychotic symptoms.

- Bipolar affective disorder: manic or depressed ± psychotic symptoms.

- Severe depressive episode with psychotic features.

- Recurrent depressive disorder; current episode severe with psychotic symptoms.

Organic

- Drug-induced/alcohol.

- Temporal lobe epilepsy.

- Other (systemic lupus erythematosus, third ventricular tumour, etc.). Again, only state these if you really are considering them in the differential diagnosis for this particular case.

INVESTIGATIONS

Physical

Think out in advance which investigations are **appropriate** for each illness.

"These could include . . . "

CBC/ESR/B12/fol.
RF?/LFT/TFT/gam
urine

- Bloods. State which and **why**. These could include full blood count (FBC), plasma viscosity (PV), renal, liver, calcium, sugar, vitamin B_{12}, folic acid, VDRL (Venereal Disease Research Laboratory) test and thyroid function tests. Know what these are done for and the relevance if they reveal an abnormality.

- Urine drug analysis.

- Electroencephalogram (EEG).

- Computed tomography (CT).

- Blood alcohol levels, etc.

Use common sense! Say what you do **in practice**.

Psychological

Tests such as psychometric testing, mood rating scales, etc., may be indicated.

Social

Do not neglect these. They are a very important part of good psychiatric practice. Because of this, you need to mention them.

> - *"I would obtain the old notes and read them."*
> - *"I would speak to a relative, with the patient's consent."*
> - *"I would speak to the ward staff and ask does the patient eat, sleep, socialise, etc."*
> - *"I would consider other sources of information: Consultant, GP, etc."*
> - Self-monitor; drinking or eating diary.
> - Specialised reports can be requested if appropriate (e.g. social report or psychometric testing).

Say **why** you would pursue each of these courses of action.

MANAGEMENT (only for Part II)

This is summarised fully in the next chapter.

PROGNOSIS

State *your experience*, not just papers. Consider:

1. The classical prognosis of this condition.
2. Specific features of this patient which affect it in this case:

- Previous history.
- Response to medication.
- Compliance with treatment.
- Social supports.
- Characteristics and strengths of the patient.
- Skills acquired.
- Degree of intelligence and willingness to work.

SUMMARY

Sometimes people find it helpful to remember this style of presenting the clinical case by using the mnemonic:

I   Overall **I**mpression
D   Differential **D**iagnosis
J   Your **J**ustification for and against each potential diagnosis
A   **A**etiological factors (the three Ps)
I   **I**nvestigations (physical, psychological and social)
M **M**anagement
P   **P**rognosis

REFERENCES

[1] M. Gelder, D. Gath and R. Mayou, *The Oxford Textbook of Psychiatry*, 2nd edn, Oxford Medical Publications, Oxford, 1989.
[2] G. W. Brown and T. O. Harris, *Social Origins of Depression*, Tavistock, London, 1978.

Chapter 8

Presenting to the examiners

Chris Williams and Peter Trigwell

There will usually be two College examiners there when you present your long clinical case. Do not be worried if a third examiner (the external examiner) is sitting in the background. He or she is present merely to record whether the performance of the examiners appears reliable and valid. They will make no contribution at all to your final mark, which is decided by the other two examiners alone.

PRESENTATION TECHNIQUES

- Go in and act confidently.
- Do not say your name. State your **examination number** when asked (have it written down).
- Shake the examiners' hands if they initiate this.
- Smile and try to remember the examiners' names.
- Look professional and act competently.

- Be polite but do not come over as too eager to please.

- Make eye contact with both examiners as you start presenting, **and** subsequently.

- Avoid looking at the floor if you don't know something. If the examiners enquire about something that you have forgotten about: *say that you would normally have enquired about this, and say why it would be important **in this case***.

- Try to appear human by showing (positive) aspects of your personality.

- Don't shuffle the papers too much.

- Be clear and confident.

- Remember, the examiners know very little about the patient.

- **Be interesting!**

It is also important to be adaptive and flexible. **Carefully consider any suggestions the examiners make** to you about diagnosis, etc. Do not reject this out of hand, but show that you can consider the relative evidence for and against a particular diagnostic possibility. If what they say throws you, remember (and tell the examiners) that all you can comment on is the evidence that you found at interview. The patient may have changed since the history was written for the examiners, or the patient may now be partially treated or have relapsed. It is quite reasonable to say this, and this further shows that you are thoughtful and clinically astute. Also, remember the clinical effects of medication on the mental state.

DIFFICULT QUESTIONS IN THE LONG CASE

There are certain areas and questions that may come up which cause candidates unnecessary anxiety. They should not, as they can be tackled in a straightforward and systematic way.

1. The psychodynamic formulation

Sometimes an examiner will ask you to present a psychodynamic formulation of your case. Do not be thrown by this. You already have all the information that you require to answer this in your case history. Consider the person's:

1. **Mother and father**.
   Their relationship with each.

2. **Personal history**.
   Important issues/factors that stand out as being psycho-dynamically relevant.

3. **Defence mechanisms**.

- Have any (e.g. projection, denial, etc.) been used in the past?

- Look for **continuity of these defence mechanisms over time**.

4. **Features at interview**.

- This may include avoiding painful issues, or crying when particular issues are touched upon.

- Consider both conscious coping mechanisms and unconscious ego defence mechanisms.

5. Keep your formulation **simple**. Address it to the **specific patient**. Say why these features are important, e.g. in considering treatment:

"It would be important therefore, to consider these factors in treatment . . . "

2. "Describe this person's personality"

Again, this is not as difficult as it may seem. You must comment upon three areas:

1. In my experience, is their personality **normal or abnormal**?

2. If it is abnormal, do they cause themselves or others to **suffer**?

   (i.e. **Do they have a personality disorder**?)

3. If they do have a personality disorder, **which one is it in ICD 10**?

   To do this well, you need to **know** the criteria. **Learn them**. If none of the criteria are fully present, say so:

   "They do not exactly fulfil the criteria for any specific personality disorder. However they show aspects of certain ICD 10 personality disorders, including . . ."

INTERVIEWING IN FRONT OF THE EXAMINERS

During the clinical examination in both Parts I and II of the exam, you will be required to interview the patient in front of the examiners for approximately 5–10 minutes. The purpose of this is to allow the examiners to gauge:

- Your professionalism (confidence, safety and consideration for the patient).

- Your manner with the patient (tact, empathy and self-control). **Some examiners are irritated if you are too familiar with the patient**. You should always refer to them as Mr, Miss, Ms or Mrs, etc., and not address them by their first name.

- Your clinical skills as a psychiatrist (listening skills, objectivity, interview skills).

- Your ability to elicit and demonstrate psychopathology (goal-directed, phrasing of questions).

Many candidates find this a most stressful experience. It is rarely practised beforehand, and hence is a potential "weak-spot". As with any task, you can improve your performance through practice. Practise this part of the exam under examination conditions at least five times in advance. It may be possible to do this within the setting of ward rounds, but it is better to do it as a separate exercise. You need to discover your potential weaknesses, and work to improve them. Ask yourself:

- *"Do I come over as a professional doctor with good clinical skills?"*

- *"Do I show myself to be a warm, genuine listener, and at the same time can I take charge and direct the clinical interview?"*

- *"Can I work efficiently to gather specific information in a clear way?"*

- *"Which clinical symptoms do I find the most difficult to phrase questions about?"*

- Develop your own style and way of asking clinical questions.

You can improve each of these areas by practice. Practice leads to confidence and increased skill. It will also help to reduce the high levels of arousal that may reduce the effectiveness of your performance.

The examiners want to know if you can **control the interview**, ask clinical questions competently and **structure your time** to complete the task in the time allocated, whilst being professional and polite to the patient. You must also come over as being genuine. If you have problems with being warm and empathic do not overcompensate. This will appear false. You are far better off in this circumstance if you adopt a professional manner that is polite and not brusque.

Typical questions the examiners may ask you with the patient present

There are certain questions which can be answered well in 5–10 minutes. You may be asked to:

1. Gather facts.

- *"Take a full alcohol history."*
- *"Assess the suicide risk."*

2. Elicit symptoms.

- *"Can you ask about their ideas concerning cleanliness and try to show whether this reflects an obsessional illness or not."*
- *"You mentioned that at times they feel threatened by those around them. Can you please ask a little more to try and decide whether these ideas are delusional."*

3. **Confirm or disconfirm a diagnosis**.

- *"You mentioned earlier that it is possible the presentation may be caused by schizophrenia. Can you ask the patient more to try and examine this diagnosis in greater detail."*

4. **Carry out specific tasks**.

- *"Test the cognitive state of the patient."* (Or specific parts of this.)

- *"Can you test the orientation and short/long term memory of the patient please."*

Techniques

- Remember you have done this many times before.

- **Write down the questions the examiners wish you to cover**. If you are uncertain, ask for clarification.

- Set up the chairs that you and the patient will sit in so that they are at about 90 degrees, and a comfortable distance apart, reflecting your knowledge of good interview technique.

- Introduce the patient to the examiners.

- Show the patient to their chair.

- **Set the scene to the patient in front of the examiners**. Show that you are aware that this is

stressful for the patient as well. Try to help
the patient relax and put them at ease. Say
something like:

*"**Thank you** for coming in. It's **important** for me
to be able to talk to you in front of the examiners
for the purposes of this exam. Try to **relax** if you
can, because it's me who is under the spotlight
today, rather than yourself, OK? I want to ask
you **some questions which we've covered
already**, but if you'll just bear with me it will only
take **about 5 or 10 minutes**. Is that all right? . . .
Thank you. Well I'd like to start by asking you
. . . "*

- Always address the patient as Mr, Miss, Ms or
  Mrs X. **Never** use their first name.

- Make sure that you cover all the questions that
  you are asked to. Maintain momentum.

- Start from first principles. **Do not** refer to things
  the patient has already told you during your
  first meeting with them. This can cause you to
  ask them very leading questions, and shows
  poor technique; e.g. *"I would like to ask you
  one or two further questions about the problems
  with checking that you mentioned earlier."*

- Make it obvious to the examiners which
  questions you are answering. If you feel that you
  are "stuck" on an area, you can always move
  on and justify your decision later to the
  examiners.

"I have a number of things that the examiners want me to cover in only a few minutes. Do you mind if we move on from this area?"

- Try to **ask open questions first**, followed by more closed questions.

- If the examiners have asked you to check whether a particular symptom is present do this quickly and efficiently. For example, if you are asked to elicit and see if a belief is a delusion (i.e. a fixed, false and unshakeable belief), then you must try to demonstrate that this is the case in the face of argument and evidence to the contrary, or that it is based on delusional evidence.

- At the end of the interview, **thank the patient again** and shake them by the hand. Do not be too deferential, just polite. Show them out of the room.

At the end of the interview, after the patient has left, the examiners may ask you what you noticed, and whether you were happy that you elicited the information adequately. **Be honest**. They may also ask whether any new information has been unearthed which may influence your differential diagnosis or management. If this is the case, say so, again showing that you are able to assess and integrate new information.

Don't worry if the patient does not give the answer that you expect. Ask again in a different way. If at the end of a reasonable selection of questions things still seem unclear, move on. You can always be honest and tell the examiners if they ask you whether you felt you carried out an adequate assessment. If you feel you have not been able to confirm or refute the symptom, then you could say:

"I didn't feel that based on the replies that the patient gave I would want, at the present time, to say that there was evidence of the symptom. I would want to spend more time with them to check this further."

The Present State Examination (P.S.E.)

One of the worries that candidates often have is *"How should I ask appropriate questions?"* There are no absolutely right or wrong ways of asking questions. It is best to develop a style that is your own, which you remember and feel comfortable with. Make sure you know how to ask about the presence of:

1. Psychosis:

- Hallucinations (auditory, visual and somatic).
- Delusions (paranoid, grandiose, hypochondriacal).

2. Other symptoms:

- Depersonalisation/derealisation.
- Worry.
- Anxiety.
- Panic attacks.
- Obsessions/compulsions.
- Hypochondriasis.
- Suicidal ideas.

Most people find that it is the "psychotic" questions which are the hardest to phrase, as well as those asking about depersonalisation. Practise these in your everyday history-taking. If you are uncertain how to phrase the questions, look at questions used in the "Present State Examination" The most up-to-date version of this is contained in the *Structured Clinical Assessment in Neuropsychiatry (SCAN)* assessment[1]. These start with "open" questions; they have been widely used in clinical research settings and have been found to be reliable. Because of this, their use cannot be argued with by your examiners. Many previous candidates have found these standardised questions very helpful.

Typical PSE questions include:

1. Delusional mood.

- *"Have you ever had the feeling that something odd is going on that you can't explain?"*

- *"What is it like?"*

2. Depersonalisation.

- *"Have you felt recently as if the world is unreal, or only an imitation of reality, like a stage set?"*

- *"Have you felt that you yourself are not a real person, not really part of the living world, like an actor playing a part?"*

3. Delusions of reference and persecution.

- *"Have you felt that people are unduly interested in you, or that things are arranged so as to have a special meaning?"*

- *"Does anyone seem to be trying to harm you (trying to poison or kill you)?"*

SUMMARY

- **Write down** the areas you're asked to cover by the examiners.

- Be confident and take charge (you've done it all before).

- Arrange the chairs.

- Show the patient in.

- Introduce the patient to the examiners.

- Show the patient to their seat.

- Have a "speech" prepared in advance about what you have been asked to do.

- If possible use PSE questions. Obtain a list of these before the exam and learn the most "difficult" ones (e.g. depersonalisation).

- Elicit what was asked for. **Open questioning** is best, leading onto closed questioning.

- Thank the patient again. Show them out and go with them. Be polite and courteous.

- Return with calm confidence!

REFERENCES

[1] The World Health Organization, *SCAN Structured Clinical Assessment in Neuropsychiatry*, Geneva, 1992.

Chapter 9

The long case: clinical management for the Part II exam

Chris Williams

You want to show the examiner that you are competent, safe and sensible. It is important to say basic principles first even if they seem obvious:

> - *"I would admit for a period of assessment."* (if appropriate)
>
> - *"I would want to treat each of their problems in turn . . . "*, etc.

STRUCTURED MANAGEMENT PLANS

Treatment of depression

1. **Psychological**.

- Supportive psychotherapy.

- Cognitive therapy of depressive cognitions.
- Treat hopelessness in particular.
- Build relationships, encourage hope and trust.

2. Physical.

- Tricyclic antidepressants.
- Selective serotonin reuptake inhibitors.
- Electroconvulsive therapy (ECT).
- Lithium.

You would always give information to the patient about delayed responses and possible side-effects in clinical practice, hence you should say this in the exam.

3. Social/behavioural.

- Offer encouragement.
- Rally supports (family/friends).
- Activity scheduling: begin to do things again, bit by bit.
- Giving permission to have time off work, etc., can help significantly.
- Reintroduce fun things that the patient has stopped doing.
- Discuss with relatives and friends about management options, if appropriate, and with the patient's consent.
- Support carers.

Treatment of anxiety

1. **Psychological**. Do simple things first:

- Education. Tell the patient about anxiety and its mental, somatic and behavioural effects.

- Reassurance.

- Consider cognitive behaviour therapy. Identify and challenge unhelpful thoughts/ worries.

Other approaches are more strictly psycho-educational or behavioural:

- Teach relaxation skills, etc.

- Look for avoidance and treat by **exposure and response prevention**.

- 2. **Physical**. Try to avoid tablets if possible, but you may wish to consider:

- Tricyclic antidepressants.

- Beta blockers if there is a sympathetic nervous system focus.

- Low dose neuroleptics.

- Avoid benzodiazepines.

Stress to the patients that the drugs you are giving aren't addictive, and discuss side-effects. This will increase the chances of compliance.

3. Social/behavioural.

- Tackle stressors/problems, debt/housing, relationships, in collaboration with other members of the multidisciplinary team.

- Exercise may help.

- Reduce caffeine and alcohol if taken to excess.

Treatment of schizophrenia

1. Physical.

- Neuroleptics (oral, intramuscular, depot) may be given at the lowest effective dose (to reduce side-effects), for only the required time (to reduce the risks of tardive dyskinesia).

- Anticholinergics (e.g. procyclidine) are only given **if necessary**.

There is little evidence to support the use of other treatments, with the exception of electroconvuls-ive therapy (ECT) in treatment-resistant cases (and even then, this tends to be used only rarely).

2. Psychological.

- Supportive counselling.

Consider family interventions for **high expressed emotion**. This means you must say something about the role of emotional arousal in schizo-phrenic relapse. The following areas have been found to be important:

- Critical comments.
- Emotional overinvolvement.
- Hostility >35 hours per week.[1]

Interventions may include:

- Education of carers (e.g. the illness, symptoms, etc.).
- Support groups for carers.
- Family therapy.

In chronic treatment-resistant schizophrenia consider offering the patient ways of distracting themselves from the "voices". This can include the use of:

- A personal stereo.
- Earplugs.

3. Social/behavioural.

- Supportive help.
- Look at strengths/weaknesses.
- Encourage independence.
- Occupational therapy/rehabilitation.
- DRO (Disablement Resettlement Officer)/ sheltered work.
- **Support carers**.

Think about where the patient is best placed to live (hostel/hospital/flat/warden, etc.). State that you would discuss the options with the patient and their family. Say that you would do this in a multi-disciplinary context, and that you would consider the Care Programme Approach.

REFERENCES

[1] C.E. Vaughan and J.P. Leff, The influence of family and social factors on the course of psychiatric illness. *British Journal of Psychiatry*, **129** (1976) 125–137.

Chapter 10

Patient management problems

Chris Williams

Patient management problems (PMPs) occur in the Part II examination only. They are set by a second pair of examiners, and will take place at the same centre and on the same day as the long case.

It is important to **practise PMPs**. Many candidates find them surprisingly difficult, simply because they have not become familiar with the technique. In fact they are very simple, because all you have to say is what **you** would do in practice. You have been solving similar problems whilst "on call" for the last few years. Be sensible and safe, and you will pass.

You will be expected to answer with a level of knowledge which is reasonable for someone of Senior Registrar level. Do not be put off if the question is put to you by an examiner who you fear may be a specialist in the area of the question they ask. For example, if you have never done child psychiatry do not be put off by questions such as *"How would you treat urinary incontinence in a child by using the Star chart method?"* All that will be expected is for you to have a reasonable overall level of knowledge, and to understand the general principles involved. You will also probably have an ally in the other examiner who is unlikely to be of the same speciality!

PMP TECHNIQUES

It is essential to be **systematic and organised** in your approach to answering PMPs. It is quite reasonable to make some brief notes as the examiners ask you the question. Have a small piece of paper or a notebook available to write on if you wish to do so.

It is important in answering PMP's **not to restrict** your answers so that you only answer one part of the question. It is easy to make the mistake of answering on only one area or aspect of the problem, thus going down a "blind alley" and running out of things to say. **Keep your thinking broad. Be flexible.**

Try to avoid a lengthy pause. You can **gain thinking time** by saying what the main thrust of the question involves (thinking out loud). Comment upon:

1. **Issues**. What are the main issues raised by the question?

- Safety/risk issues.

- Diagnosis and management.

- Any Mental Health Act/Common Law issues?

- Patient issues (compliance, etc.).

2. **Information**. Do you need any more information? Where from?

- To make the diagnosis.

- To decide on treatment.

- Impact on the patient: what has he/she stopped doing because of the problem?

- Impact on other people (e.g. carers).

Remember to consider **psychological** and **social** aspects of diagnosis and treatment as well as **physical** ones (e.g. effects on the patient, their family and work). What are the benefits and risks of treatment?

*"This question involves a number of different **issues**. It raises the importance of being sure of the original diagnosis, the need for a full assessment, and also the difficulties of treating those with treatment resistant depression . . ."*

*"In this case I would wish to gather further **information** in order to clarify the diagnosis. I would talk to . . . in order to find out . . ."*

This has the advantage of showing the examiners that you can pick out the **key points** quickly and have a firm grasp of the essentials of care.

Another way of helping you gain valuable thinking time is **to talk yourself into the situation** and allow the examiners to again realise that you grasp the key features of the case:

"If I was asked to go and see this patient in casualty, I would begin thinking about how to manage the case on the way there. I would first go to the Medical Records Office, look up and obtain his old notes and quickly read them in order to find out more information. I might also phone the ward where he had been an in-patient and see if any of the nursing staff knew him . . ."

If you do not know an answer, say where you would go for appropriate and sensible advice. For example, if you do not know what drugs you can safely prescribe in pregnancy, it is reasonable to say *"I would contact the pharmacy and Drug Information and ask for further information."*

If the examiners appear to strongly disagree with you, be prepared to consider other possibilities. Feel able to discuss other diagnostic or treatment options. **Never get into an argument**, but if you feel that you are correct, you should review with the examiners the reasons for and against each of the possibilities, and the reasons why you wish, for the time being, to stick to your first decision. Always show that if more information became available, or the person changed, that you would be willing to reconsider.

The principles of effective answering of PMPs are illustrated in the following example. Variants of this type of question are commonly asked in the exam.

Example:
Treatment-resistant depression

"A 65-year-old man has been weepy and depressed for 3 months. He has lost a significant amount of weight and there is marked anhedonia. He has been treated with dothiepin for the last 8 weeks and continues to be very low in mood. He has begun to express ideas of hopelessness and is feeling suicidal."

The examiners will ask questions such as the following. These may be given consecutively to test the depth of your knowledge as you answer, or may be asked together all at once.

- How would you manage this patient?

- Would you make any change of medication? If so, what would you do and why?

- You make all these changes and he continues to be unwell. How would you manage him now?

Spend about 5 minutes answering this question by jotting down your answers on a piece of paper. Try to be **organised** as you answer. What are the **main points** you need to cover?

Possible components of the answer

1. Is the diagnosis correct?
   In a 65-year-old-man with weight loss, perhaps there is a hidden physical disorder (such as cancer). Has this been excluded?

*"I would want to confirm that the diagnosis
actually is depression. I would do both a full
psychiatric history and also a detailed mental
state examination. I would examine the person
physically and send off appropriate screening
bloods for physical disease. In particular, I
would request a full blood count to check for
anaemia, and thyroid function tests to exclude
thyroid disorder. If any other physical tests are
warranted, I would request these (e.g. a chest X-
ray in a smoker).*

2. Gather more information to make sure.

*"I would also obtain the **old notes** and read
them. It would be helpful **to talk to an informant**, with the patient's permission. I would also
like to get a clear description from **nursing staff**,
etc., of how the patient is during the day to see
if their behaviour is consistent with a diagnosis
of depression."*

3. Check current and past management.

- Ask other obvious questions: *"Are they actually
taking the dothiepin?"*
- Are they taking an appropriate dose?

*"I would want to know if they are taking the
tablets at an adequate dose. I would increase
the dose up to the stage where side-effects are
noticed. Although conventionally around
150 mg of tricyclic are prescribed for most*

patients and this is viewed as a "standard" dose, this varies (e.g. in older people). If tolerated, higher doses may be safely prescribed in younger adults, possibly with ECG monitoring.

One important focus of this question is "How do you treat resistant depression?" This is a classic and often repeated PMP. A clear and concise summary is contained in *Dilemmas and Difficulties in the Management of Psychiatric Patients.*[1,2]

One approach might be to:

- Increase the dose of antidepressant to a high level.

- Augment with lithium.

- If there is delusional depression, add a neuroleptic. This also acts to increase tricyclic antidepressant levels.

- If the person is on a tricyclic there is **little sense** switching to another tricyclic.

- If the person is on a SSRI, switch to a tricyclic and increase the dose.

If this doesn't work, either:

- Add ECT.

- *or* Switch to a monoamine oxidase inhibitor (MAOI).

Know about **washout periods** for these switches and also for the switch from a SSRI to a tricyclic.

Do not neglect to mention **maintaining factors**. It is easy in a question such as this to only mention physical approaches to treatment. Abnormal personality and ongoing social and relationship problems are potent maintaining factors for depression. These would need to be addressed. Sometimes adding cognitive behaviour therapy can make a difference by challenging the "negative cognitive triad" of self-defeating thoughts that may be maintaining the depression. Beware of hidden physical disease. Finally, if the person is still depressed, referral to a psychiatrist who has a different theoretical orientation to your own may be helpful.

The concept of **secondary gain** may some-times be useful to consider, *but* its mention is **fraught with danger** in exams. It should only really be mentioned if there is clear evidence that it is a contributing factor to the lack of progress.

The examiners may then either go on to another PMP, or add a further stem to the current question which will introduce a fresh angle to the problem:

"The gentleman is admitted to the ward, and unfortunately then commits suicide whilst there by hanging himself one night. He was supposed to be on close nursing observation at the time and hanged himself whilst in the shower."

- What would you do in these circumstances as the Senior Registrar? Your Consultant is on holiday.

Again, spend a few minutes thinking about how you would answer this question.

When it comes to the second part of this question (i.e. the problem of the suicide), say what you would do in practice. This would include:

- Informing and discussing the case with the Consultant who is covering for your absent boss. You would do this in practice, so say so.

- Informing the hospital managers of the death.

- The Police and Coroner would of course have to be informed.

- A major emphasis should be on support and help both for colleagues and for relatives.

- There should be an attempt to gather information about the events leading up to the death and this should be clearly documented.

- Meeting with all the nursing staff, and the Charge Nurse or Sister in charge would be important.

- Disciplinary actions may be an issue; however, this would be instigated from within the management aspects of the unit. Support for staff, and clear communication with relatives is paramount. It would be important to avoid blaming anyone.

It is important to remember that there is **no absolutely "right" answer** to any PMP. There are a number of ways of answering. What matters most is that you are seen to be safe and sensible.

Do not begin to answer each question in exactly the same way. This will annoy and frustrate the examiners.

The other PMPs, which are given in Appendix 2, illustrate the importance of **not panicking** when you are asked a difficult question. You know what you would do in these circumstances. It is merely a matter of **organising and structuring** your answer. If you do not know the answer, or are confused by the question, **be honest** and say so. It is far better to move on to an area where you are scoring marks than to stick with a topic where you gradually disappear into a hole that is self-created.

The answers that we have given are deliberately overinclusive. You might not be able to provide this much information in an exam setting.

SUMMARY

Remember:

- What are the main **issues** (patient, Mental Health Act, etc.)?

- Do you need further **information** (physical, psychological and social)?

- Management (physical, psychological and social).

- Treatment benefits and risks.

- Do not panic!

- Be sensible and safe.

- Say what you would do in practice.

- Be divergent in your thinking and avoid going down a blind alley.

- Organise your answer clearly.

- Do not be dogmatic. Show that you are flexible and will consider the evidence for and against a range of diagnostic or treatment options if this is appropriate.

- Where appropriate, say that you would seek advice or information from others with more experience in that area.

- If in doubt act **safely**. The key questions the examiners are asking are: *"Is this person **safe**, **sensible** and in touch with the **standard practice** which reflects a reasonable level of care?"* Make sure you are!

- What would a real Senior Registrar do? Do it!

RECOMMENDED READING FOR THE PMP EXAM

We suggest that you read the following for the PMPs and also for the clinical exams. They are excellent books for helping you decide what to do in difficult clinical situations, and how to manage a wide variety of practical (and common) clinical problems. **Read them if you have time**.

[1] K. Hawton and P. Cowen (Eds), *Dilemmas and Difficulties in the Management of Psychiatric Patients,* Oxford Medical Publications, Oxford, 1990.
[2] K. Hawton and P. Cowen (Eds), *Practical Problems in Clinical Psychiatry,* Oxford Medical Publications, Oxford, 1992.

Chapter 11

If at first you don't succeed . . .

Kevin Appleton

Not everyone passes the MRCPsych. Approximately 45% of candidates are successful at each sitting. Many people have sat the exam one or more times previously. Failure will be experienced by a large number of candidates at some time whilst trying to pass both Parts of the MRCPsych exam. I was such a person. This short section is dedicated to those people who may have a similar experience to me at some time. There are those who work long and hard, apparently covering all the topics thoroughly, but who still fail. This is a most disheartening experience and can cause a myriad of feelings including upset, and anger.

It is difficult to alleviate the sense of disappointment and exhaustion that follows the receipt of your application forms for the next attempt and condolences from the Chief Examiner. At this stage try to send off the form to **request feedback on your performance as soon as possible**. It is easy to be so fed up that you feel you never want to do the exam again. You may adopt an attitude somewhat akin to "learned helplessness". Failure will trigger off many thoughts that will convince you that Beck's negative cognitive triad is an accurate model of depression. You will feel pessimistic about yourself, the world and the future. You will begin to make negative predictions, and have the most catastrophic thoughts about the exam or your career. As with all such thoughts, they are both unhelpful and inaccurate.

Sending off for feedback can actually help challenge these beliefs. It can show you that **you are not bad at every part of the exam**. Realising this can be quite encouraging. You will have done better on some parts of the exam than others. This is useful information, because it shows you which areas of your performance you need to change. Receiving this feedback can help you feel that you've made the first step toward slaying the dragon when you next meet it (a bit like sending your sword off to be sharpened)!

Next is the difficult task of giving the bad news to others. Everyone wants to know if you passed, but no one wants to ask you. Your colleagues may study you intensely from a distance to pick up clues (drooping shoulders, dishevelled appearance) before deciding whether to sit with you at lunch. Some people do genuinely wish to hear all about it and may allow you to offload your sorrows. For others, try using a brief but positive sound-bite. Alternatively, consider wearing a black tie for several days. Humour can sometimes be a great healer. You could even have a lapel badge saying *"DON'T ASK!"*

At some stage you do need to accept the fact that failing an exam is a kind of bereavement. You need to give yourself time to recover before starting again. Try to be good to yourself, get plenty of sleep, and go out and do some of your favourite things. Do something different which is fun (and non-psychiatric). A short holiday away, or booking onto a course you have always wanted to do can be useful. Life is for the living and your brain and body will need a well-earned rest. There may also be practical matters that have been neglected during the intense revision and that need to be caught up with. Dealing with these will take your mind off the exam and put things in perspective. Family and friends may have had less of your time and attention recently, so take the opportunity to remedy this. They need to have you back for a while and you need their support and encouragement. Try and move your focus away from just the exam; in the long term, failing the exam will not seem that important, and may well be a time that helped you learn more about yourself and your priorities in life. No one in their right mind would choose to fail, but if it happens it isn't the end of the world. Worse things do happen, and a quick break to watch the news will remind you that on the world scale of events failing the MRCPsych exam is actually not so bad.

You will have to try to work out exactly what did go wrong in your performance, and start to plan a strategy for another attempt. At a fairly early stage you should decide whether you are going to re-sit at the next opportunity or wait 6 months or more. This decision will have to be based on a number of factors. These may include practical matters such as pregnancy, house moves or any other foreseeable events that might make it just too difficult to give enough time to your revision. If possible, applying to re-sit soon is probably the best thing to do, for two reasons. First, it helps you maintain momentum. Even if you take 6 or 8 weeks off from learning after the last exam, your previous revision will be relatively fresh in your memory. You can use this as a firm foundation to build on. Secondly, there is only a short window of opportunity where you are allowed to apply for the exam. If you miss it, you will not be able to apply for the next sitting. If you are in doubt it is often best to apply and secure a place. For many people motivation to work comes back slowly with time, and this can be accelerated by having the focus (and financial commitment) of a booked exam. If you change your mind later, you can always choose to withdraw prior to the exam without this being counted as an attempt. There will be a financial penalty for doing this, however, as outlined in the College application forms.

The initial feedback from the College will tell you which part of the exam you have failed. The later feedback (which you have to request on a form sent in the "fat envelope") may not arrive until a few weeks before the next exam. Do not wait until you receive this to go to see your clinical tutor, consultant, or other helpful persons who can help you at your next attempt. If you don't already belong to a study group this may also be the time to get together with three or four like-minded people who intend to take the exam at the next sitting. These groups can be a great source of support, encouragement, shared knowledge and learning.

After failing Part II, I felt that, although I possessed a lot of theoretical and practical knowledge about psychiatry, I had not used or communicated this well in the exam itself. My second attempt involved a much greater emphasis on technique, after attending the Leeds MRCPsych Examination Technique course which gave rise to this book. Much useful work was also done in study group gatherings. With a pile of textbooks on the floor and plenty of chocolate biscuits and coffee we would go through hundreds of MCQs, SAQs and PMPs. This helped to focus my learning on exam-relevant information, and I would recommend it.

On a philosophical level it is helpful to try to see positive aspects of failing the exam:

- You will have the theoretical framework of the exam firmly fixed in your mind for next time.

- It will give an opportunity to improve learning and study skills.

- Failure might also be an experience that brings understanding and insight not otherwise gained.

- Keep on trying!

"With perseverance a blade of grass can split rock."

(I Ching, The Book of Changes).

Appendix 1

What are Mind Maps® and how can they help with the exam?

Kevin Appleton

You will already be aware of your strengths and weaknesses when it comes to learning for exams. You will probably use techniques which you have (successfully) used over the years. Successful techniques allow you to structure, organise and integrate new information with the information that you already know in order to make learning meaningful. This is important because, particularly with the Part II exam, it is a practical impossibility to read through everything again in the few days before the exam. It is important to focus on key facts, so that these may be concentrated on in order to reduce the amount of reading you have to do when the work is revised.

Common and effective techniques for helping you reduce the quantity of information you have to learn include writing short summary notes or using highlighter pens to focus in on key facts. Another less common approach is Mind Mapping. This is not an approach that everyone will find intuitively appealing; however some people find this approach to be a very helpful way of organising and learning information.

Mind Maps® are colourful, branching pictures or diagrams that

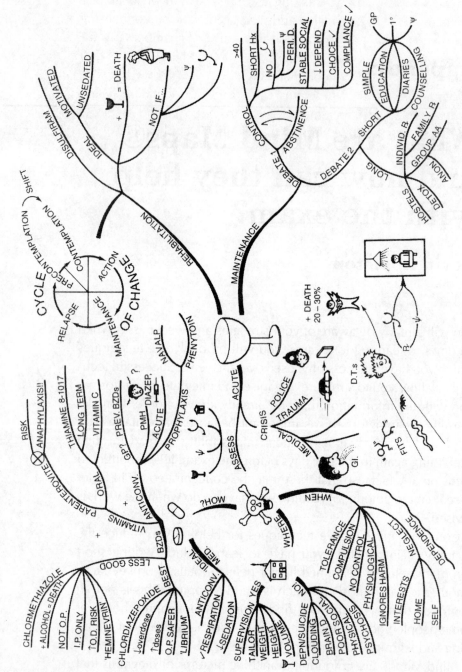

Mind Map®1. Alcohol assessment, complications and treatment.

can help your memory, thinking and organisation of ideas and information. They can make study more efficient by condensing more facts onto a single sheet so that very large amounts of information may be revised very quickly. In Mind Map® 1 the assessment and treatment of alcohol addiction is covered, together with the ways that alcohol problems can lead to presentation to the medical services. To maximise the effectiveness of Mind Maps® it is necessary to produce your own so that each subheading of the Mind Map will trigger off associated pieces of information in your own memory. If you had Mind Map® 1 in front of you during either an essay, SAQ, PMP or clinical viva, you would be able to answer most questions on this topic.

Mind Maps® work by increasing the cross-connections and associations of stored information in memory. They use images or key words to anchor information and to trigger associations. It is possible to hold entire Mind Maps® in visual memory by this method – and they are fun to use, making learning more enjoyable and revision less tedious. By using different modes of memory storage (e.g. factual, visual and colour), they increase the modalities and ways in which information can be remembered, whereas linear text uses only one such modality.

HOW TO CREATE YOUR OWN MIND MAPS®

It is better to draw Mind Maps® across the horizontal axis of the page, as the structure spreads out better this way. Start with a central image or icon. Recalling this from visual memory will trigger your recall of the whole map. Next, arrange main headings or key words around this from the centre of the page. Subheadings, lists and further details can then be added to each branch.

One heading or icon (e.g. head injury, as in Mind Map® 1) will come to represent, in your own mind, many other additional responses (subdural, penetrating, etc.). These act as anchors for surrounding text and help you to recall this additional information efficiently. Well-organised information should result in an aesthetically pleasing map, whereas poorly organised information will

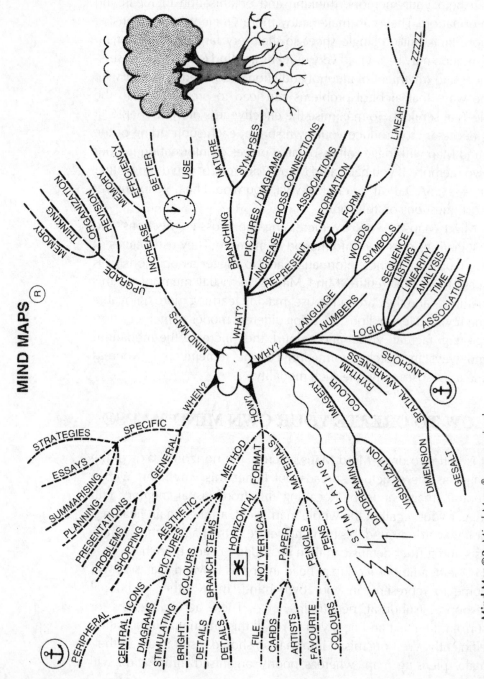

Mind Map®2. Mind Maps® summarised.

look a mess and will be less well recalled. To structure the content clearly on paper means that it must also be structured clearly in your mind, so that drawing out the diagram is itself an effective means of revision. This is illustrated by Mind Map® 2, which summarises the use and production of Mind Maps®. You will see that the key elements of the linear text you are now reading are clearly and concisely summarised on one sheet of paper. This is both information rich, and very quickly read. If this is the case for this section of the book, could it also be the case for your exam revision?

Because Mind Maps® can be used to summarise large amounts of information into a manageable form, the information can be reviewed very quickly just before the exam, maximising the recency effect. In the 48 hours before the written paper I was able to review the entire syllabus, which I had summarised into Mind Maps®.

A full account of the use of Mind Maps® is given in *The Mind Map Book.*[1,2]

REFERENCES

[1] T. Buzan and B. Buzan, *The Mind Map Book*, BBC Books, London, 1993.
[2] The Buzan Centre Ltd, 37 Waterloo Rd, Bournemouth, BH19 1BD. Tel. 01202 533593 Fax 01202 534512
® Mind Map is the Registered Trade Mark of the Buzan Organisation.

Appendix 2

Practice patient management problems

Chris Williams

The following patient management problems (PMPs) illustrate the range of questions that you may be asked as part of the Part II clinical examination. You will find it useful if a colleague asks you the questions under exam conditions. Try to be concise and organised in your answers. Ask for specific feedback on your performance, or tape your answers so that you can listen to the content and style of delivery at a later time.

PMP 1

A 35-year-old married woman comes to Casualty after being found unexpectedly by her mother after taking an overdose of 60 paracetamol and a bottle of wine. You are called by the Casualty Officer after she refuses to have a washout or take Ipecac. She says that she is going home and that she doesn't care if the tablets harm her. You discover from her mother that her husband left her for another woman 3 weeks ago and that since then she has been upset and weepy.

- The Casualty Officer wants you to section her so that medical treatment can be offered. What do you do?

- Would you be forced to let her go if she insisted on going?

- She now gets up and makes a run for the door. What actions might you consider in this circumstance?

PMP 2

A 32-year-old lady comes to see you in out-patients. She has known bipolar affective disorder which has been successfully treated with lithium carbonate for the last 4 years. She currently has a stable mood, and is quite happy taking the lithium. At the clinic appointment she says that she and her husband want to start a family.

- What would you advise?

- She now decides to stop the lithium and becomes pregnant. How would you treat her manic relapse in pregnancy?

- How would you manage her if she relapsed soon after birth?

- What are the risks of medication. What treatment would you advise?

PMP 3

You are called to a medical ward to see a 55-year-old man who had a myocardial infarction 3 weeks ago. He is now "profoundly depressed" according to the House Officer. After making a suitable assessment you are clear that the diagnosis is clearly a depressive disorder.

- How would you manage this patient?

- What antidepressant might you use?

- If he didn't get better, what other treatments may you use?

- This gentleman has now suffered a stroke. Would a SSRI (selective serotonin reuptake inhibitor) be safe in a stroke?

PMP 4

You are on-call in the hospital. You are phoned by the GP who tells you that a 29-year-old gentleman who is known to have a long history of schizophrenia is about to be brought to the ward by Police after he has smashed up his flat. He has been seen by the Senior Registrar at home, and at present is saying that he will come into hospital. On previous admissions to the same ward there have been major problems because of violence and overarousal as a result of his illness.

- How would you manage this case?

- What would you do in anticipation of his arrival?

- How would you approach the interview with him?

You are later called to the ward. He has become acutely aggressive and is being held to the ground by three staff nurses. He is shouting and angry and says that people are trying to kill him.

- What would you do?

PMP 5

You see a bus driver in the out-patient clinic. He presents with low mood and nightmares which began when he knocked over a little girl 6 months ago. He is still off work, and is very anxious about returning to his previous occupation.

- What issues would you bear in mind during the assessment?

- If the diagnosis is one of post-traumatic stress disorder, how would you approach each of his problems?

Index